PENGUIN BOOKS

The Ice Diet

Peta Bee is a health and fitness journalist who writes for *The Times*, the *Sunday Times* and the *Irish Examiner*, as well as numerous other publications. With degrees in sports science and nutrition, Peta likes to probe the evidence behind latest fads and trends and her work has won her numerous awards, including the Medical Journalists' Association's Freelance of the Year (twice). She has appeared widely on television and radio and is the author of six other books, including *Fast Exercise*, the 2014 bestseller co-written with Doctor Michael Mosley. She lives in Berkshire with her family, who have long forgiven her for turning down the heating.

The Ice Diet

PETA BEE

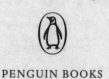

PENGUIN BOOKS

PENGUIN BOOKS

Published by the Penguin Group
Penguin Books Ltd, 80 Strand, London WC2R ORL, England
Penguin Group (USA) Inc., 375 Hudson Street, New York, New York 10014, USA
Penguin Group (Canada), 90 Eglinton Avenue East, Suite 700, Toronto, Ontario, Canada M4P 2Y3
(a division of Pearson Penguin Canada Inc.)
Penguin Ireland, 25 St Stephen's Green, Dublin 2, Ireland (a division of Penguin Books Ltd)
Penguin Group (Australia), 707 Collins Street, Melbourne, Victoria 3008, Australia
(a division of Pearson Australia Group Pty Ltd)
Penguin Books India Pvt Ltd, 11 Community Centre, Panchsheel Park, New Delhi – 110 017, India
Penguin Group (NZ), 67 Apollo Drive, Rosedale, Auckland 0632, New Zealand
(a division of Pearson New Zealand Ltd)
Penguin Books (South Africa) (Pty) Ltd, Block D, Rosebank Office Park,
181 Jan Smuts Avenue, Parktown North, Gauteng 2193, South Africa

Penguin Books Ltd, Registered Offices: 80 Strand, London WC2R ORL, England

www.penguin.com

First published 2015
001

Every effort has been made to ensure that the information contained in this book is accurate.
Following a diet is not always the right decision for every person, and should in any event be
undertaken only by those without underlying health problems. If in doubt, please consult your doctor.
Neither the publisher nor the author accept any legal responsibility for any personal injury or other
damage or loss arising from the use or misuse of the information and advice contained in this book

Set in 12.5/14.75pt Garamond MT Std
Typeset by Jouve (UK), Milton Keynes
Printed in Great Britain by Clays Ltd, St Ives plc

ISBN: 978-0-718-18074-4

www.greenpenguin.co.uk

Contents

Introduction

Hear the word 'diet' and what springs to mind? Self-imposed starvation and stomach-grumbling? Calorie restriction and energy slumps? It's fair to say that most of us have encountered the downsides of dieting at some stage in our lives. In the last two decades, my job as a health journalist has introduced me to almost every fashionable new diet and exercise regimen to hit the headlines. Much of what I have seen has left me cynical.

I've discovered that the diet and fitness industries too often base themselves on false and flash-in-the-pan promises with short-term appeal, often restricting food choices to such a degree that there's barely anything left to put on your weekly shopping list. What's hot to eat (or avoid) today will invariably not be the thing that promises to make you thin tomorrow. And evidence backing the claims for many trendy eating plans and detox regimens is often alarmingly scant.

My background in sports science and nutrition left me with a burgeoning sense that weight loss comes down not just to what we eat, but when we eat it and how we live. In a nutshell, that's what led me to the science that underpins the Ice Diet. So what does it involve? Well, what you won't get on this diet is hungry. Neither will you be asked to crunch on ice cubes, take freezing-cold daily baths or generally subject yourself to temperatures that a polar bear would find challenging.

You will be eating delicious daily meals that provide a balance of macronutrients (fat, protein and carbohydrate), as well as all the vitamins and minerals you need to stay healthy. And you will lose weight. Not just because of the changes to the food you are eating, but by embracing Nature's very best fat-burning mechanism: cooler temperatures. We all feel like hibernating when it's cold. But science has proven that most of us are now warm to a fault and it is impacting our waistlines and our health. By reversing the habit, you really can transform your body for the better.

Sounds incredible? When I first came across the alleged benefits of exposing our bodies to cooler temperatures – not just outdoors, but within the home – I too was highly sceptical. I'd been asked to write an article for a national newspaper that would involve me taking part in a trial being conducted by scientists at the University of Nottingham's Queen's Medical Centre. Professor Michael Symonds and his team got me and other subjects to plunge our hands into a bucket of cold water before checking on high-tech thermal imaging cameras to see how our bodies responded. After just a few seconds of cold-water immersion, calorie burning was boosted. It was a revelation and triggered a strong urge for me to find out more.

There was something else that helped to sway my thinking. As a young university student in the north of England, I'd noticed that during the autumn and winter months, repeatedly and without exception for at least the ten years that followed, I lost weight without trying. Not a colossal amount, but enough to be noticeable. It was, I remember thinking, as if my body was consuming itself to stay warm. I could literally feel myself gobbling up extra calories simply to protect myself against the seasonal drops in temperature.

Being students, we were short of money and consequently, relative to today, short of food. We went out – exercising, to the pub, to lecture theatres – just to stay warm. It was little more than a hunch, but over the years I felt a certain pleasure at the arrival of the first annual cold snap, in the knowledge that I would at least be leaner for a few months as a result. It took on more significance in recent years when I realized that my seasonal weight loss, while still evident, was slowing down.

Whereas I'd found it easy to drop half a stone without much effort in my cold student and early career days, the scales were much less kind once I hit my forties. Age and the slowing metabolism it brings almost certainly had a role to play, I deduced. But I also knew that my lifestyle was considerably warmer. I'd become more deskbound, more prone to cranking up the heating and far less tolerant of cold in general. Only when I visited Professor Symonds's labs and began investigating the links between healthy diet, cooler living and fat burning did the coin drop: the three really are inextricably linked.

Since then, I have interviewed dozens of leading experts, trawled through hundreds of scientific papers and spoken to people who really believe that by eating well and by doing their utmost to activate good fat and inject coolness into their lives, they have transformed their waistlines and their health for the better. And I've discovered that ice is undeniably cool. Many A-listers and elite athletes are already using coolness in the belief that it will boost calorie burning and fitness. From Daniel Craig, Usain Bolt and David Beckham to Demi Moore, Halle Berry and Jennifer Lopez, a regular dose of cool temperatures has become a way of life. Celebrity trainers like Romana Braganza, who works with Jessica Alba, and Jon Denoris, whose clients include Rachel Stevens and Whitney Port, prescribe cold exposure for calorie burning.

What I've discovered along the way has radically changed the way I live. And I am lighter, less prone to illness and fitter as a result. What's more, my family is also more brimful with vitality and wellness. Now it's your turn. In *The Ice Diet*, you too will discover the mounting and convincing scientific evidence that how you live is affecting your weight; that Nature intended us to eat well and to experience cold, not to be permanently stifled by warmth, and that our bodies respond positively to mild 'thermal stress'. If you embrace only a few of the principles outlined in the pages that follow, you will be a healthier, and undeniably cooler, person for it.

PART ONE

1 Ice Power

Dieting can be brutal. It can leave you tetchy and tired, unhappy and hungry. Not this one. From the offset I would like to stress the good news: that a leaner, lighter new you can be achieved on a daily intake of nutrient-dense foods with rich flavours. You can eat deliciously well and still shed weight. What matters is not just how much you eat, but how often. And also how well your diet and lifestyle work in tandem to naturally turbocharge your fat-burning capacity.

Later on in the book, you will learn precisely how food deprivation is not essential for shedding pounds. On the contrary, you will discover that a wealth of tantalizing and satisfying meal plans and recipes await. Before that I need to explain how and why you will be able to eat so well. So, first comes the science bit . . .

Cool History

Our ancestors didn't have central heating and thermal base layers to stay warm. They didn't inhabit the hermetically sealed boxes we now call our homes and offices. There were no coffee chains luring them with hot, creamy drinks and steaming snacks, all promising to keep them toasty at the first sign of a winter chill. High-tog duvets were unheard of. So were duck-down jackets, handwarmers and snow boots. Against the odds, perhaps, they survived.

Part of our evolutionary survival was the human body's ability to adapt to variations in temperature from occasionally mild and even warmer than we experience today to bitterly cold, and to food scarcity and the physiological demands of hunting for something to eat and then conserving that energy in case no calories were available in the forthcoming days. Over seven million years, our genes became primed to withstand challenges that seem alien to the environment in which we find ourselves living today.

Food is in constant and overwhelming supply. And we are nearly always warm. Even compared to our grandparents, we have become a coddled generation, so that when winter comes we rarely encounter seasonal icy blasts. We have entered what some scientists have called a state of 'thermal monotony'. So accustomed are we to pervasive warmth that we barely register how hot our lifestyles have become. Our homes are warmer and so are our places of work. We exercise, shop and eat in warm environments. We wear ski jackets on mild autumnal days and drive around in heated cars when it's too cold to walk. Our inner temperature gauge is rarely challenged and, when it is, we just head indoors and turn up the thermostat. With the flick of a switch, we are artificially warmed; we never have to acclimatize to the plummeting temperatures outside.

I grew up in Birmingham in the 1970s and 1980s where we lived in a three-bedroom semi with windows that rattled and allowed draughts to whistle through. There was no double glazing and, like all of our neighbours, we had no central heating. I remember that during one particularly harsh winter our toothpaste froze in the tube overnight. In each of the two downstairs rooms there was a single three-bar gas fire that my mother would crank into action only when it got 'too chilly'. Such occasions were few and far between. Looking back, those fires were rarely switched on. We were told to put on a thick sweater if we were cold and were given an extra blanket at night if our feet were still ice blocks an hour after going to bed.

What strikes me as I think back to my childhood is not just how much colder we were, but that it didn't matter. Nobody knew any different and we dealt with seasonal changes in temperature by warming ourselves naturally. Our bodies adjusted. We were sent outdoors to play so that we'd feel warmer when we came inside. We drank cocoa and hot drinks. We moved about more. We didn't think about cold as a form of discomfort, but as a passing inconvenience. It would be better by spring.

Hot Houses

Quite how much our homes are hotting up is staggering when you look at the statistics. The average home is at least 5 °C (9 °F) warmer than it was thirty years ago and we spend in excess of £4 billion on keeping our homes cosy.[1] On average we heat our homes up to 23 °C in the winter, but often much hotter. One third of people bask in homes heated up to 25 °C and one in twenty lounge in a tropical 30 °C.[2] Government-backed surveys show that nine out of ten householders admit they simply turn up the heat if they feel a bit cold rather than the cheaper and infinitely healthier option of adding a layer of clothing.

Traditionally, the big switch-on of central heating occurs in mid to late October when the clocks go back. But we have become a nation of softies. Pre-autumn chills at which we once wouldn't have flinched now trigger a mass turning-on of central heating and firing up of the boiler. Companies like npower say they record a 65 per cent increase in demand for gas in early to mid-September, even during weeks of late summer sunshine.[3] In 2013, 45 per cent of people turned on their heating at the beginning of September when temperatures averaged 14 °C. It has been attributed to a 'faux winter' effect in which we feel colder than we actually are: temperatures might drop by as little as 0.25 °C but we perceive the dip as more significantly chilly because we are so used to being warm.

A Hot House Can Make You Yawn

If you find yourself yawning at work or home more often than you used to, the chances are it is not because it is contagious or because you are bored but because your brain is too hot. Researchers at the University of Vienna in Austria found that the only reliable and significant predictor of yawing was high temperatures. Even factors like how much sleep a person had the night before did not seem to influence how often they yawned as much as temperature.[4]

Does It Matter That We Are Warm?

Of course, there is an argument that our heated lifestyles are a form of progress. We are comfortably warm, so why change? It comes back to the way our bodies and genes are programmed to adapt to mild cold stress. An in-built response mechanism forged centuries ago ensures that we not only acclimatize to cooler conditions but, as we will see more of in later chapters, we thrive in them. They keep us lean and ward off waistband thickening by releasing hormones and increasing beneficial substances within our systems that boost calorie burning. Cold helps us fight fat more effectively.

It is no coincidence that with rising indoor temperatures has come a corresponding rise in obesity. In a review of what they call the 'Metabolic Winter' phenomenon, one group of esteemed scientists from Harvard Medical School and the University of New South Wales summed it up in a nutshell: 'Obesity and chronic disease are seen most often in people and animals (pets) they keep warm and over-nourished.' We carry with us, they wrote, 'the survival genes for winter', but we never need to use them.[5] The upshot? Warm living is making us weigh more; we are literally too hot for our health.

As a scientific theory, it is fast gaining pace. Researchers began to suspect a link between warm surroundings and weight gain around a decade ago, but it was a paper published by a group of British scientists in 2011[6] that first looked specifically at whether indoor central heating, in particular, could be a factor in fatness. What the researchers observed is that as central heating has become more commonplace, so weight problems have risen.

Whereas previous generations – even our grandparents – would heat only the main living areas and not the bedrooms or bathrooms, we now heat the whole house, often with under-floor heating systems as well as several radiators in a room. No longer having to adjust to different temperatures as we move through a house leads to a sort of 'thermal comfort zone' that affects the way we burn up energy. Scientists in that early paper went as far as saying that heating has a significant impact on energy balance and an impact on body weight and obesity. Since then others have reached the same conclusion: that our hot houses and offices are contributing to our ballooning waistlines.

What Happens When We Get Cold?

We shiver, of course. Shivering thermogenesis, as scientists refer to it, is our response to being exposed to frigid temperatures. As muscles contract and expand around vital organs in short bursts, the body generates heat and boosts energy expenditure by as much as five times the level in a resting state. In the short term it does its job well and protects against hypothermia.

But there are other emerging benefits of shivering episodes that are far more exciting as they help to unlock some of the mystery surrounding the obesity epidemic.

Shivering sparks a series of hormonal and chemical changes deep within the body that alter fat cells and boost metabolism in much the same way as an hour-long workout. Remarkably, that's what investigators from the US National Institutes of Health (NIH) found when they invited healthy men and women to a laboratory on three different occasions for a study.[7]

During one of their visits, the volunteers were asked to complete a high-intensity exercise session by cycling hard on indoor exercise bikes until they were exhausted. On another occasion, they rode at a more leisurely pace for an hour. Both of these workouts took place in a room maintained at a comfortable 18 °C. On their third visit, however, the room temperature was dropped to a chilly 11 °C and the men and women were asked to wear light clothing and to lie on a bed for half an hour. By the end of the thirty minutes they were noticeably shivering – and understandably so.

Throughout the trials, the researchers were taking blood tests and muscle samples to find out how the subjects' bodies were responding to the various ordeals. In particular they were looking for changes in levels of a substance that is now considered a key part of cold-induced calorie burning: brown adipose tissue (BAT), brown fat, or – as it's become better known – good fat. Unlike the kind of white fat that settles stubbornly as a paunch or saddlebags, good fat burns calories like a furnace. Rodents and babies – not good shiverers – are born with it to keep them warm and until a few years ago it was widely believed we didn't store it in our bodies after childhood. But studies that have emerged since 2009 have proven that to be untrue. Good fat stores have been detected in humans of all ages. Some have more than others and, as we will see in Chapter 2, we have the power to activate it, to turn on its full calorie-blasting potential. Shivering, it seems, is one of those triggers. When we are cold, this metabolically active tissue launches into action to warm us up.

When the NIH scientists analysed their data they found that levels of hormones known to create brown fat were markedly higher in blood samples after the exercise bouts – but they were just as elevated when the volunteers lay quietly and shivered. In a nutshell, the calorie-burning effects of an hour-long cycle can be achieved by lying still in a cold room.

The Pre-Shiver System

A downside to burning calories through shivering is that it is unpleasant. Downright miserable, in fact. Even with the promise of a leaner and lighter body, who wants to be exposed to that level of discomfort? Not me, for sure. Shivering is debilitating. We get nothing done when we are trembling with cold.

So, here's the good news: we don't have to live in a human fridge to lose weight. Exposing ourselves to less extreme temperatures can also burn calories by the bucket-load. This comes down to a process that takes place within the body pre-shiver, when you feel cool but not freezing. As your body prepares to keep you warm, it produces heat internally before you start to quiver with the effects of the cold. Medically known as non-shivering thermogenesis, it activates good fat and powers up calorie burning in much the same way.

It's such a new area of study that researchers are still trying to pinpoint the precise mechanisms that unleash this pre-shiver response. Skeletal muscle and tissues are thought to be involved, but what's clear from the evidence is that it 'contributes significantly to total energy expenditure'[8] and everyday fat burning. How much energy is burned varies from person to person. Some children and the elderly respond poorly to being cold and don't pre-shiver much at all. But for the average young adult through to those in their fifties and sixties, it is estimated the internal fuel burn can be boosted by one third when we sit, work or walk in a cool environment.

What does this mean for fat loss? You will find out more when we delve deeper into the nitty-gritty as we progress through the book, but suffice to say the outcome can be pretty impressive. Just two hours a day spent in a cooler-than-average environment with a temperature of 17 °C, led to a significant increase in good body fat in one group of men.[9] And in an experiment with seventeen hardy volunteers,[10] who spent six hours a day for ten days at 15 °C dressed only in shorts and T-shirts, what Dutch scientists found was fascinating. Conditions were undeniably chilly, but over the ten days they got better at generating heat without their bodies resorting to shivering. In other words, they acclimatized and switched to pre-shivering mode, their metabolism improved and they burned more calories. Not that the Dutch scientists advocated freezing as you watch TV. They suggested that 'mild cold training' in which rooms are heated to a comfortable 18–19 °C and slightly cooled every so often by turning down the thermostat by 2 °C produced calorie-burning increases of up to an impressive 6 per cent daily.

A Bedroom Tale

I've always been a fan of a cooler bedroom. I find it helps me to sleep comfortably. Conversely, hot and stuffy hotel bedrooms are my worst nightmare. I toss and turn, desperately looking for windows that open more than the locked inch to which they are set for safety reasons. My preferences were seen as quirky when I first met my partner, a confirmed hot-houser at the time. But a degree of persuasion and careful acclimatization over the years mean he is now, still somewhat begrudgingly, in the cooler bedroom camp. Which, I guess, is fortunate considering we both have to share the same sleeping environment.

Lo and behold, scientists recently provided just the backing for my long-held hunch that a bedroom can be too hot. Aha, I said, waving the wad of a published study that confirmed what I'd been trying to tell him. The research, part of the ICEMAN study (Impact of Chronic Cold Exposure in Humans),[11] hinted that lowering the thermostat could augment the many well-documented values of sleep on health by subtly transforming good brown fat stores as we are in a slumber. The result? Our metabolic health and calorie-burning capacity could be accelerated not just while we lay snoring and dreaming, but even into daylight hours.

To test out the theory, five healthy volunteers were asked to sleep in climate-controlled chambers at the headquarters of the US National Institutes for Health (NIH) for four months. During the day, the men worked and exercised as normal and ate meals that were provided as part of the study to make sure each had the same calorie intake. Then they returned to the laboratory chambers at 8 p.m. each evening, where they would sleep in hospital-issue pyjamas under light cotton sheets.

For the first month, the experience wasn't too arduous. Their bed chambers were maintained at a neutral temperature of around 24 °C (75 °F), considered comfortable by most people. In the second month, bedrooms were cooled to 19 °C (66 °F), not frigid enough to cause shivering but a level the researchers suspected would stimulate good brown fat into action. In month three of the study, the controlled heating was re-set at 24 °C (75 °F) to ensure their body responses to the chillier temperatures were cancelled out. During month four, the heating was turned up to a positively toasty 27 °C (81 °F) to see what happened when they slept in relative warmth.

Researchers kept track of blood sugar and insulin levels, but also tracked the daily calories that were burned and the amount of good fat that was active. Results were fascinating. There were marked changes in the men's bodies after the four weeks of sleeping in the cooler 19 °C (66 °F) rooms and, most significantly, during this time they almost doubled their concentrations of good fat. They also burned extra calories throughout the day and there were positive changes in their insulin sensitivity, meaning their ability to control blood sugar improved.

Conversely, when the bedroom heating was turned back up to 27 °C (81 °F), the metabolic improvements were undone and the effects reversed. The amount of good fat in the men's bodies dropped to such an extent that they had less than when the trial started. Professor Francesco Celi, one of the researchers, said he is a fan of cooler bedrooms and that turning down the thermostat at night is an easy and effortless way to stay lean. Remember, his subjects were ordinary young men and 'just by sleeping in a colder room they gained metabolic advantages'. How easy is that?

Scourge of Central Heating

Ironically, the more control we have over the thermostat, the more control it has over us. It dehydrates us, dries us out, saps us of energy, makes us more prone to dribbly noses and infections and, of course, means we rarely allow our good fat to be activated indoors. Then we get landed with a huge bill for the privilege. While boosting weight loss might be your primary reason for turning down that dial, it is not just your waistline that will benefit. As temperatures rise when heating is turned up, it dries out the atmosphere and the body responds in different ways, none of them particularly desirable.

Many people find they develop cold-like symptoms, a result of chemicals released as part of the body's response to the rise in temperature. Known medically as Vasomotor Rhinitis, it causes blood vessels to pump so that more blood reaches the nasal area. What follows is sneezing, an uncomfortable itch and a runny nose. Because central heating also dries out the moist membranes of the lung, it renders the body less able to fight off viruses and other infections.

Hotter indoor living environments have been linked to a rise in skin problems such as eczema, as well as lethargy, poor concentration and disturbed sleep. A report by Allergy UK[12] revealed that when the colder months arrive, closing doors and windows and turning up the heating creates a breeding ground for house dust mites and mould. Around 50 per cent of people who are allergic to mould say their condition worsens when the heating is on. All the more reason to open a window and stay cool.

Baths and Showers

It's hard to believe that in 1951, two-fifths of UK homes were still without a bath or shower. Yet research at the University of Lancaster into the culture of bathing and showering reveals that less than a century ago, a weekly bath was considered perfectly adequate, and even our grandparents thought it acceptable to wash thoroughly just a couple of times a week. Now, we think nothing of showering once, twice or even three times a day, before and after work or going out and after the gym. I am as guilty of this obsessive cleansing as the next person, often totting up two or three submersions in a twenty-four-hour stretch.

What's concerning is that the water we use is getting ever hotter. Water runs out of hot domestic taps at 70 °C, which is far too hot for bathing in and can easily cause injuries. Ideally, when you have a bath or shower, the water should be slightly warmer than your body temperature, which is, on average, 37 °C. Most of us like it to be hotter than that, preferring to immerse ourselves in temperatures of 39 °C or higher. A few years ago a government minister prompted public outrage when he said he was considering regulating the maximum temperature of domestic baths and showers by fitting thermostatic mixing valves, which would fix the maximum temperature at 46 °C, in all new homes. Although the plans never came to fruition, they are perhaps not as ridiculous as they sounded at the time.

Understandably, there is environmental opposition to using as much hot water as we do. And it's only going to get worse as industry forecasts predict a five-fold rise in the total amount of water used for showering in the years from now up to 2021. But there are reasons beyond water wastage to switch to cooler washing. For men, too many hot baths have been shown to cut fertility. Sperm counts in five out of eleven men with fertility problems soared by 491 per cent after they stopped soaking in hot baths or using hot tubs for a few months. Sperm are known to develop best in cool conditions, which is why the testicles are situated outside the male body, and researchers from the University of California confirmed a few years ago that 'wet heat' could damage fertility by 'overheating' the sperm.[13]

Dermatologists fear that our habit for such regular washing in hot water is stripping the skin of essential oils that keep it supple and moisturized. Every time you take a bath or shower, you're sloughing away at your skin's structure. Soap and hot water dissolve the lipids in the skin and scrubbing with a flannel or loofah only hastens the process. The more baths and showers you take, the more frequently this damage takes place and the less time your skin has to repair itself through natural oil reproduction. In short, daily dousing with hot water combined with harsh soaps can strip the skin of its oils, resulting in dryness, cracking and even infection.

Cooler washing might also boost your mood. As we've seen, our ancestors were frequently exposed to brief changes in temperature and, throughout evolution, our own bodies have remained primed to thrive under the same physiological stressors. Without this kind of 'thermal activity', researchers are beginning to think that our brains can function inadequately, leaving us prone to depression. What's really interesting is that early trials have indicated that a cold bath or shower could simulate the kind of thermal stress needed to prevent mood swings.

How this works is fascinating. Exposure to colder water is known to activate the sympathetic nervous system and to increase blood supplies of endorphins (feel-good hormones) to the brain. With a huge number of cold receptors in the skin, a cold shower in particular is thought to send overwhelming quantities of electrical impulses from peripheral nerve endings to the brain, boosting our mood in the process. When a group of subjects were asked to take a 5-minute lukewarm shower followed by 2–3 minutes of cold water (20 °C) once or twice daily for several weeks as part of preliminary studies, the treatment had a significant anti-depressive effect.[14]

Keep Your Cool at Work

As one of the growing army of home-workers, I find one of the advantages is that I can blast myself with fresh air, open a window when I am weary or just step outside when I feel that I am getting cabin fever. I have long preferred to work in slightly chillier conditions during the winter months, feeling it makes me more productive.

Millions of office workers don't know when the sun is shining and have no idea how warm or cold it is outside much of the time. Some are cooped up in surroundings where the nearest window is a corridor away. Does the heat of our workplace make any difference? One study[15] tested whether work output and thinking power improved or deteriorated as temperatures were raised or lowered. Volunteers were first asked whether they preferred working in a warmer or cooler office and then split into groups accordingly. Each group was given a set of thinking tasks on a computer and asked to complete them in three different office spaces – the first heated to 25 °C (77 °F), the second a cool 15 °C (59 °F) and the third set to 20 °C (68 °F).

Results showed that no single temperature out-performed the other when it came to correct answers in the tests. But all subjects had better scores when they undertook the task in the room of their preferred temperature. Those who had said at the start of the study that they liked an office to be cool did better at 15 or 20 °C. Those who liked it hot excelled in the warmer environment. What it shows us is that, provided we acclimatize to having the thermostat lowered, excess warmth offers no advantages when it comes to promoting efficiency and productivity at work. If we learn to like cooler rooms and are given time to adjust to them accordingly, then we will work just as well in those conditions.

Ice Man

During the course of researching this book, I've come across a number of leading metabolic experts and physiologists, sport scientists and biologists who really do walk the walk when it comes to keeping cool. All, in their own way, are waging a war on society's increasing and unnecessary hunger for warmth by starting with themselves, putting into practice what they have discovered from research.

Among the most inspirational is an Alabama-based man called Ray Cronise. Ray is a former NASA scientist who discovered, through experiments on himself, how shunning hot temperatures can accelerate weight loss. His name cropped up with such frequency when I began researching coolness that I knew I needed to track him down. Wherever I looked, he was there: on blogs and websites, in university research teams and in papers published in esteemed scientific journals.

When we eventually spoke for the first time, I realized we were kindred spirits when it comes to the cold. We are both convinced that being overly warm spells trouble for a society's waistline. We have since swapped scientific papers and spoken at length about what works and what doesn't when it comes to shedding pounds. Ray has opened my eyes to new areas of thinking and has proved inspirational in many ways, not least through his own story. It is remarkable and will most likely strike a chord with many of you, as it did with me. By his own admission, Ray was overweight. Pounds had crept on here and there during his twenties and thirties. 'I don't know how, but I woke up and I had swelled from 170 pounds to 230 pounds,' he says. 'I might have actually weighed more, but I stopped keeping track of it and I rarely wanted to measure anything.'

We all know that feeling – hiding away the scales because we don't want to know the worst. Ray tried diet after diet and found they worked up to a point, but then the weight (or at least some of it) settled back on. He wanted to get his 5-foot-9-inch frame back down to a healthy 180 pounds, but it was an uphill struggle. A turning point came when he was watching a documentary about the Olympic swimmer Michael Phelps in 2008. It revealed that, even by an athlete's standards, Phelps ate an enormous amount of food to fuel his training efforts. On a daily basis he needed to pack away 12,000 calories, more than Ray was consuming in a week. It puzzled him how a man would need that much energy just to maintain his physique and strength. Yes, Phelps was fit and extremely active and his training regime took an enormous calorie toll in itself. But there had to be something more, Ray thought. Other top sports people didn't need that much food, despite their equally arduous physical demands. So what was different? Phelps was, of course, spending much of his time – up to four hours a day – in water. And not particularly warm water at that, but pools heated to only around 26.6 °C. It struck Ray that this daily exposure to cooling was having a dramatic effect on Phelps's energy stores, that his body was burning an extraordinary amount of calories just to stay warm and maintain his core temperature of 37 °C. What if Ray could simulate that effect by other means? Would the weight drop off?

It's fair to say that the notion became something of an obsession for Ray. 'I wanted to get to the bottom of how he was burning so many calories,' he told me. 'I wanted to really understand why it seemed so difficult for me to lose a couple of pounds and yet I could easily gain a couple in a weekend.' Ray deduced that his body had forgotten what it was like to be cold, that he needed to reintroduce that sensation into his life and see if it somehow triggered him to lose weight. It was a shot in the dark and he wasn't sure whether his self-experimentation would pay off. But it was an intriguing enough theory to give it a go.

Initially, he dived in at the deep end, sometimes into icy waters. In those early days, Ray took cooling to extremes to see how his body would react. He recalls sitting outside on a particularly chilly day (0.5 °C) wearing nothing but shorts – no shoes, socks, top or hat. He shivered uncontrollably for what he reckons was probably the first time in his life. After a time, it was beyond uncomfortable. His hands and feet hurt, his ears, nose and face burned, so he went inside. In the weeks that followed he took cold showers and went on 1–2-mile 'shiver walks' wearing just a T-shirt, gloves and earmuffs on his upper body and shorts or light trousers on his lower half.

He drank a gallon of ice water every morning and slept under light sheets rather than a heavy duvet. He ate the same number of calories as he had been doing (12,000 a week over six meals a day) and kept up his usual exercise programme. Ray lost 9 pounds (2.7kg) in the first week. After six weeks he had tripled his previous weight-loss rate with a total loss of 27 pounds. Being a scientist, he didn't stop there. 'Most people going through a mid-life crisis will invest in a sports car,' he says. 'For me it was a top-of-the-range Italian calorimeter that I put in a room next to my kitchen so that I could measure how energy was affecting my body in every way.'

In the intervening years Ray has tested and re-tested his cooling methods until he has reached what he believes to be the optimal approach. It is far less extreme than he originally expected it would need to be. His body has gradually acclimatized to downward shifts in temperature so that it can tolerate bouts with the thermostat set to

15 °C–17 °C, the temperature used in many scientific studies to boost good fat and calorie burning. He finds that 'contrast showers' – in which fast bursts of cold and warm water are interspersed for several minutes, as opposed to freezing-cold prolonged drenching – are enough for weight loss. 'It's important for people to realize that they don't need to join the polar bear club and start taking ice baths or ice showers,' he now says. 'It doesn't have to be intolerable.' He doesn't shiver miserably. And he has lost (and kept off) the weight he set out to shed.

I've shared this story because it demonstrates probably better than any other how quickly science evolves. When he started his self-experimentation, it's fair to say that Ray was considered a maverick, a slightly crazy ice man with crackpot theories about how we should live and what was causing so many people to be overweight. How things have changed. Ray's hunch that the obesity epidemic was down to more than the food we eat is rapidly gaining credence. As more has become known about the effects of cold since he first started his experiments and as research has validated many of his previously untested hypotheses, Ray has risen to the higher echelons of science.

He is invited to speak at top medical conferences about his cooling methods and theories, and was one of the co-authors of the 'Metabolic Winter' paper I mentioned earlier, written with Dr David Sinclair, a researcher at the Harvard Medical School Department of Genetics and the Department of Pharmacology at the University of New South Wales, and Dr Andrew Bremer, a renowned endocrinologist who currently works at the NIH as director for Type 2 diabetes prevention and kidney disease medical officer. Ray writes a fascinating blog[16] about his cool approach to life which is a must-read if, when you have finished this book, you want to know more.

My point is how quickly his theories, which seemed unlikely at the offset, have been validated by the world's leading experts. Ice power and the potent effects of cooler living are undoubtedly the hottest topic in weight-loss research.

How Cold is Too Cold?

Shivering temperatures, ice baths and a dip in freezing water are not my thing. Neither, I suspect, are they yours. As we've discovered, our bodies have an amazing ability to adapt to cold temperatures over time. We acclimatize well, within reason. But our tolerance to the cold varies. So how cold is too cold? Generally, hypothermia is a risk for adults at temperatures below 0 °C or below 15 °C in water. Young children are less able to thermo-regulate in the cold than adults and there is a risk of chilling generally in the elderly. People taking certain medications, including beta-blockers, sometimes report a lower tolerance to the cold and there's some evidence that certain drugs block the pre-shivering response.

It's a fallacy, though, that women are more susceptible to the cold than men. It's been widely speculated that men should have a higher tolerance because of their greater ration of body mass to surface area and the fact that their bodies generally have more heat-producing muscle. But the science isn't clear cut. And several studies have shown the opposite to be true – that women are less susceptible to hypothermia. Women do tend to have colder hands (I can vouch for that, mine being icy all year), but that's now thought to be a positive as it means they are better at directing body heat to protect vital organs.[17]

The general consensus is that a healthy adult's cold response, particularly to immersion in chilly water, depends more on their body size and percentage of body fat than on gender.[18] And, of course, it is never good to get too cold. We are not penguins or seals. Our core temperature is 37 °C because our body generates heat. Subjecting it to sub-zero conditions is asking for trouble. Don't dive into icy waters, literally or figuratively; make the transition from warm to cool for optimum benefit.

What It's Done for Me

Keeping ourselves coddled is now so normal that initially it is shocking to suggest we do the opposite and turn the thermostat down. I can't say I relished the prospect when I first read about it. During my childhood and teens I inhabited an altogether cooler environment. But in the intervening years, much like almost everyone else, my life had heated up. I had hot baths or showers on a daily basis. I was as guilty of hiking up the heating as the next person – at home or in the car, and when I was working.

I'd go out running in more layers than I needed only to find myself sweltering after the first few minutes.

What made me make the switch? As I outlined in the introduction, it boiled down to two factors: the memory of being cold and the way it made my body feel or react, and the emergence of engaging science that proved there was more to the links with fat loss than mere faddy speculation. Since I started making conscious attempts to live a cooler lifestyle, I've discovered some unexpected things that might further persuade you it is worthwhile:

- I feared it would be incredibly hard to do and even harder to persuade my family that being overly warm is not a good thing. This was far from the case. The key is to adjust temperatures gradually and acclimatize over time.
- I thought a cool working environment would be hellish. Unbearable. As it turns out, I am far more productive with a window open, even in the middle of winter. If I have urgent deadlines to meet I resist putting the heating on at all. However cold it is outside.
- I get more out of my workouts. I have never been much of a gym fan, although I have tried pretty much every workout and gym class going. What I've discovered since I began avoiding them altogether is how much more enjoyable exercise is when it is performed in the cooler outdoors. I find I work harder because it takes longer to reach the point of uncomfortable sweatiness.

- I sleep better. And so does my initially reluctant partner. My young son now sleeps with his window open too. We are a household converted and I feel positive that it is healthier with a breeze coming through the bedroom than sleeping in the equivalent of an airtight closet.
- I rarely get ill. And neither does my family. This is a revelation. Among his friends, my son stands alone in hardly ever succumbing to the endless round of infections that strikes during winter at primary-school age. And I can't remember the last time I got a cold. I am convinced that our cooler living is behind our boosted immunity.
- I weigh less and, since I got used to being cooler, eat less. Lethargy plays a role. When we are warm, we become sluggish and we innately crave a carbohydrate boost because we think it's what we need to pep us up. Wrong. What we really need is a blast of fresh air.

A Burning Question: How Many Calories Can Being Cold Burn?

Let's re-cap on what the emerging science has shown. How being colder – but not freezing to the point that we shiver – really can help us lose weight. As humans, we are pre-programmed to respond positively to cold temperatures. Our ancestors evolved in them and acclimatized accordingly. It means our bodies and our genes have

27

in-built response mechanisms to the cold – the activation of good fat, the burning of extra calories – all of which help us to stay warm.

By artificially heating ourselves to the extremes we do today, we have effectively switched off these survival genes. And, as a result, our daily calorie-burning tally has nose-dived. Reversing this trend to turn back on the metabolic boost through cooler living can have a dramatic effect. Published scientific studies show that turning down heating by a couple of degrees can increase calorie burn by 6 per cent. Consistent chilly living (several hours in a cool room) can see a 30 per cent rise in the amount of calories used up on a daily basis.

A more manageable and comfortable approach to cooling, though, is what suits most of us. Ray Cronise estimates moderate chilling on a daily basis can lead to a metabolic boost of around 20 per cent. That's an extra 2,800 calories a week burned by men and 2,100 a week by women. Or, as Ray puts it, the calorie-burning equivalent of running a marathon a week. Just by living as Nature intended.

In practical terms, the endpoint can be a substantial loss of weight. On average, an adult needs to burn 3,550 calories to lose one pound of fat. Just by reducing the temperature of your living environment, exposing yourself to cold blasts and embracing the seasons, you could spur your body to burn anything from 30–41 pounds of fat a year.

In the next chapter we'll look at calorie-gobbling good fat in more detail. How does it work and how exactly can the Ice Diet help to fire it into action?

2 Good Fat, Bad Fat

When you think of body fat, you probably tend to think of the yellowy-white fatty tissue that jiggles and dimples beneath the skin, that bulges over waistbands and creates spare tyres and cellulite. We know all about this kind of fat: how it stores excess calories from sugary doughnuts, cakes, snacks and crisps; how it migrates to our hips and stomachs and settles stubbornly despite our best efforts to shift it with torturous diets and exercise plans. We are well aware that too much of it leads first to obesity and that this raises the risk of us getting killer diseases like cancer, diabetes, heart disease and strokes.

But as you found out in Chapter 1, not all fat is bad. So-called brown fat or brown adipose tissue is labelled 'good fat' because of the way it works positively to fight pounds piling on. While white fat packs on to your thighs and stomach, in contrast brown fat works to burn it off. What's ironic is that just as we need it most, our lifestyles have led to our good fat lying idle.

As we've seen, our genes have a blueprint for extra calorie burning that was established by our hunter-gatherer ancestors. Today, without the need to wait for food or the need to fire up the body from within to stay warm, we have effectively turned off good fat and lost one of the crucial mechanisms that sent our metabolism soaring.

Thankfully, scientists have gone into overdrive when it comes to looking not just for ways to multiply the number of good fat cells we have, but also how to rev up its activity. In another, even newer, avenue of research, they are exploring whether it's possible to transform plain old blobby white fat cells into tissue that behaves very much like good fat, a substance they are calling 'brite' (brown fat in white).

In this chapter we will look in more detail at how good fat operates, what makes it tick and, most importantly, how science says we can spur it into calorie-gobbling mode.

Where Did Good Fat Spring From?

You might have heard about good brown fat before picking up this book, but I wouldn't be surprised if not. Even the world's leading scientists weren't aware we had it until a few years ago. They knew good fat existed. For more than three decades they had studied it in rodents and babies, both unable to shiver effectively enough to keep themselves warm, and they were aware that it acted like an inner furnace, churning up calories and churning out heat.

They also knew that around 5 per cent of a newborn's weight is brown fat, there to protect it from hypothermia, a major cause of infant death. And they had identified how it worked. Whereas white fat cells store energy as one large oily droplet, they do nothing to burn it up. Brown fat cells, on the other hand, contain numerous small oily droplets but are also packed with mitochondria, the energy powerhouses of our cells that give good fat its reddish-brown colour.

If white fat cells are the couch potatoes of the body, then brown fat cells are the Ironmen triathletes, using the mitochondria to burn up the oil and generate energy. But the general consensus was that it just disappeared when we no longer needed it. By the time humans reached their late teens and adulthood and their bodies learned the shiver response as a warming tactic, it was assumed this good fat was gone.

Three papers published in the *New England Journal of Medicine* in the spring of 2009 turned that thinking completely on its head.[1, 2, 3] Researchers carrying out PET-CT scans on subjects discovered, quite by chance, that good fat didn't disappear but, in fact, was present in nearly every adult, picked up by the scans as tiny blobs that were burning glucose at a rapid rate to produce heat.

How had they missed it for so long? It seems they simply hadn't been looking in the right place. Babies' good fat deposits are in the upper half of their spine and towards their shoulders. In hibernating rodents, it's positioned between the shoulder blades. Scientists had looked for good fat in the same areas in adults a quarter of a century earlier but spotted nothing. It turns out it was scattered more widely: in the upper back, by the collarbone, at the side of the neck and along the spine.[1]

In terms of the battle against obesity, it was the rediscovery of the decade. A flurry of scientific papers ensued and an editorial in the *Obesity Review Journal* posed the question: 'Have We Entered the Brown Adipose Tissue Renaissance?'[4] We had indeed and the calorie-burning powerhouse that is good fat is now considered crucial for weight loss.

Do We All Have It?

How much good fat we have varies. Some of us have more than others. What's important, though, is that the Ice Diet will help those with active stores of good fat to boost its effectiveness; and for those in whom it is yet to show up, it will fire it into action.

In almost everyone of normal weight or below it shows up clearly when they are exposed to cold temperatures for a short time. Younger people have more than old and women generally have more than men. Professor Michael Symonds says: 'We do know that you have less brown fat as you get older and that ties in with the other metabolic changes that occur with age. We also think there might be subtle changes in brown fat that occur around puberty.'

People with lower and more stable blood sugar levels have higher amounts of good fat than those with a sluggish metabolism, indicated by poorer blood glucose control. What's interesting is that good fat is much less visible in scans of obese people.[5] That's not to say it's not there, but one theory is that their excess body fat is insulating them to such an extent that good fat doesn't need to be switched on. Another is that the scarcity of good fat is a reason why people gain weight. Once weight is lost, it could be that good fat becomes visible in scans.

If we were to weigh out good fat on a set of scales, how much would there be? It's likely that more than half of all men and women, regardless of age, have at least 10 grams and in many cases substantially more. Women in one trial were shown to have 12.3–170g of good fat and men 0.5–42g. To put this into perspective, around 50g of ordinary white fat idly stores more than 300 calories of energy. The same amount of good fat could burn up to 300 extra calories a day if spurred into action.[6] That's getting on for a pound gobbled every week before you've even thought about eating less or going to the gym.

How Is Good Fat Measured?

Medical scanning is the only reliable way of testing your levels of good fat and how well it is activated. In the early days of the good fat revival, PET-CT scans were seen as the gold standard measuring device, but a team of British experts at the University of Warwick were the first to show good fat using MRI scans instead.[7]

MRI is being hailed as a superior method of monitoring good fat. Whereas PET scans show good fat in humans only after it has been activated by the cold, MRI technology reveals its location whether it is active or not, providing researchers with much more ammunition when it comes to developing other ways to activate it in the future.

Then there are the pioneering thermal imaging techniques such as those used by Professor Symonds in Nottingham.[8] Its appeal is two-fold: it is relatively inexpensive and is also non-invasive, making it a safe way of accurately measuring brown fat in children because there is none of the potentially harmful radiation associated with other scanning methods. Thermal imaging works by identifying hotspots of good fat under the skin by monitoring the temperature of the skin lying over the top of it. Because brown fat produces 300 times more heat than any other tissue type, heat-sensitive technology can detect it and also measure how active it is, or how much energy it is producing.

One thing is certain: as interest in good fat soars, the way we measure it will become more refined. In the future, it could be that we get 'good fat' check-ups in the same way we keep tabs on blood pressure and bone density.

How to Fire Up Good Fat

As soon as scientists rediscovered good fat and its calorie-gobbling potential, they began seeking out how best we can fire it up. New findings are emerging almost by the month and are giving a much clearer insight into how we can supercharge our bodies to burn fat. What's exciting and something of a relief if, like me, you are not keen on conventional, restrictive diets, is that many of the good-fat triggers uncovered in research and included in *The Ice Diet* are easy to adapt into our daily lives. They require us to tweak our lifestyles, not overhaul them. In practical terms, that makes it much easier to stick to long term.

It's important to remember that no single method of activating good fat is a sure-fire route to weight loss in itself. The Ice Diet is based soundly on principles of healthy eating, enough activity and the addition of good-fat boosters to maximize your weight loss. These triggers are an adjunct to sound diet and exercise, not a replacement. What I've enjoyed most is experimenting to find out what works for me. Everyone will have a favourite fat-burning trick. Part of the fun is finding out which is yours.

The Cold

Of all the ways to supercharge good fat, the most widely proven is through exposure to cold temperatures. As we have already seen, cooling your living environment can have a powerful effect on calorie burning. Thankfully, that doesn't mean taking ice baths and freezing-cold showers on a daily basis. Just living as Nature intended and embracing the seasonal changes in weather can make a considerable difference to the way our good fat behaves.

It's feasible that, by cocooning ourselves in warmth throughout the year, we are unknowingly creating another risk factor for obesity. Professor Michael Symonds and his team in Nottingham were intrigued about whether the seasonal flux in temperatures had any effect on our good fat action and recruited 3,614 patients to find out if their theories had any basis.[9] Using PET scans, they monitored both the amount of good fat and its activity in winter and summer to see if there were any differences.

Their findings were striking. Not only were the detected levels of good fat higher in the winter months, but they were also significantly more active. Colder weather clearly played a role in prompting the body to work harder to burn energy, but Professor Symonds found plummeting temperatures were not the only thing having an effect: the shorter, darker days of winter also seemed to play a part. It's further proof that getting outside when we least feel like it, when there's a biting chill and the sky above is dismal and grey, really can be good for our health.

As knowledge grows about the benefits of cool temperatures, investigators are more certain that we don't need to stay uncomfortably cold for it to be beneficial. Dr André Carpentier, an endocrinologist at the University of Sherbrooke in Quebec, kept subjects – all of whom were men – in a chilled laboratory, but not so cold that it left them shivering, a response which we have seen burns calories in itself. They wanted to look specifically at good fat.

Results showed metabolic rates increased by 80 per cent, all from the actions of a few grams of cells.[10] The brown fat also kept its subjects warm. The more brown fat a man had, the colder he could get – and the more active his good fat became – before he started to shiver. On average, the good fat burned about 250 calories over three hours.

It's worth re-capping, too, some of the other findings from the ICEMAN study,[11] the paper that found changes in bedroom temperature can influence metabolism.

Researchers, including endocrinologists from Sydney's Garvan Institute of Medical Research, were looking at the effects of altering the thermostat on the good-fat activity of healthy young men over a period of four months. Spending at least ten of twenty-four hours in temperature-regulated rooms set for the first month to 24 °C, the second month at a vastly reduced 19 °C, the third month at 24 °C again and the fourth month at 27 °C, had a dramatic effect on the men's good fat action.

During the coolest month, good fat increased by 30–40 per cent, but dropped back to baseline when the room warmed to the thermo-neutral 24 °C. At 24 °C there was no boosting effect, but at 27 °C their good fat levels plummeted to below what they were at the start of the trial. There is little doubt that keeping our cool is healthy, and that we can power up our body's internal engines considerably just by exposing ourselves to less warmth. As Dr André Carpentier put it in an editorial accompanying his published paper, cold temperatures can mean good fat is 'on fire'.

Cold Hands, Hot Burn

As I mentioned in the introduction, my interest in good fat was sparked when I visited Professor Michael Symonds in 2012 to take part in a trial he was carrying out at the University of Nottingham's Queen's Medical Centre. Michael and his team were using groundbreaking thermal imaging techniques to look at how good fat changes with age and under different conditions. Specifically,

(Continued)

they were interested in the influence of weight, Body Mass Index, food consumption and activity levels on good fat.

Previously, they had used the same thermal imaging to show that the neck region in healthy children produces heat.[8] 'There is only about 50g of brown fat in the neck region of children and it switches on and off throughout the day as it's exposed to different temperatures or if you exercise or eat,' Michael told me.

I pitched up, flustered and tired after a three-hour drive from London, and was asked to take a seat in one of the hospital labs where the trials were taking place. Using ultrasound equipment, measurements were taken of the thickness of the skin on the top of my shoulders – some studies have shown that the thicker the skin in this area, the less active the good fat beneath – and the baseline temperature of my good fat was recorded.

I was then told to sit in a comfortable position for ten minutes (without moving, to ensure my temperature fluctuated as little as possible) before plunging a hand into the bucket of water beside me. It seemed like a rudimentary experiment but the process and the outcome offered a great insight into how easily we can spur good fat into action. At 20 °C, the water was chilly but not freezing. Yet after five minutes of submersion, my hand began to numb, which was picked up by the thermal imaging camera hidden behind a screen as a startling blue. What the cameras also displayed was a distinct increase in red areas around my lower neck – a sign that my good fat stores were reacting in the way they should, producing heat and burning calories to try to keep me warm.

Professor Symonds says that my exercise regimen – I'm out-doors running or walking my dog come rain or shine, coolness or warmth, five or six times a week – has certainly helped to keep my good fat activated over the years. Combined with my relatively healthy diet, he said it was probably the reason that my weight has remained stable within half a stone for the last decade. But the experiment told me that I could do more to help my body work more efficiently. Cooler living was a simple and effective way to offset the slowing metabolism that comes with the middle years.

So what were my results? They showed that the temperature of my brown fat rose from its baseline of 34.5 °C by 0.15 °C. It doesn't sound much, but it represented a rapid increase during five minutes of cold exposure that equated to a 10–15 per cent rise in the number of calories I burned. Just by putting one hand in a bucket of water I had sent my metabolism into overdrive. If I was at all sceptical about the concept of cold being beneficial to the body beforehand, the results from Professor Symonds's experiment proved to be the turning point.

Exercise

Now we all know that exercise and dieting should go hand in hand when trying to lose weight. One relies on the other to be effective. Our metabolisms get much more of a boost when they are done in combination than when we attempt to do one of them alone.

When it came to the effects on good fat, though, investigators were struggling to find any evidence confirming that regular workouts had any direct influence. In scans, exercise didn't seem to boost the activity of the good fat that was visible beneath the skin. One reason for this might be linked to the fact that the body's core temperature rises when you work out, making it tricky for good fat to be spurred into action.

And yet, scientists had a hunch it might be working in other ways. Among the most intriguing suggestions to emerge was the idea that exercise might help us in ways we previously hadn't considered possible: by converting idle white body fat to energy-devouring brown fat, dubbed 'brite'. The possibility of this began to become apparent when investigators started looking at how activity might affect the body at cellular level. They identified several molecules that seemed to stimulate the 'browning' of white fat without the need for getting chilly.

One of those molecules, identified by Harvard Medical School experts,[12] was a new, unknown hormone released from muscle cells after exercise. This previously undiscovered hormone appeared to coax blobby white fat into behaving like good fat and, in the process, potentially reduce the likelihood of obesity, diabetes and related health problems. It had long been suspected that muscle cells communicated somehow with body fat, literally sending messages telling our blubber how to react and behave when they are active.

While working to unravel this mystery, scientists uncovered some intriguing biochemical processes, the role of the new hormone being one of them. Even the deep visceral fat that is embedded around internal organs and considered an important risk factor for disease fell prey to this browning process. It was a major discovery and the new hormone responsible was given the name irisin, after Iris, the Greek messenger goddess.

However, doubt has since been cast over the 'browning' theory in relation to exercise and many other researchers doubt whether irisin has an effect. In one of the newest and largest trials involving people, Professor Jamie Timmons of the University of London and Professor Stuart Phillips of McMaster University looked at 90 overweight people to try to determine whether white fat really is 'browned' during and after exercise. After sixteen weeks of a modestly calorie-restricted diet, the group had lost a lot of fat, but there was no apparent 'browning' of white fat cells.

Compared to the evidence linking cold temperatures to good fat, the exercise connection is flimsy. Of course, whether or not good fat is involved, exercise has many other metabolism-boosting benefits. More vigorous workouts, like cold temperatures, do produce a surge of adrenaline, which is known to activate good fat. And high-intensity exercise of short duration leads to enhanced all-round calorie burning and health improvements, making it a crucial aspect of the Ice Diet.

Food

Before we look at precisely how our diets might be able to rev up our good fat, let's remind ourselves of how our hunter-gatherer ancestors did things on the dietary front. Go back several thousand years and days could easily pass between meals. By necessity, the human body was primed for survival. It needed to prepare ahead for times when food was scarce and did so by storing excess energy in white fat cells where it was readily available as a back-up source of fuel when needed.

What helped us to survive 40,000 years ago on the Serengeti has ultimately proven to be part of our downfall, at least as far as obesity and its related health issues are concerned. Our diets have changed, while our bodies' means of dealing with them haven't much. A constant supply of food that is packed with sugar, salt and fat, and is far more calorific than that foraged for by our ancestors, has resulted in our white fat storage cells being overloaded in the extreme.

What's alarming is how overeating and the vast quantity of calories we now consume could, in turn, be causing what one eminent cardiologist has termed a 'death spiral' for good fat.[13]

Sugar and Fat

There's little doubt that overindulging on fat and sugar in the diet will eventually mean we have a larger belt to show for it. These two dietary baddies have been studied more than any other in relation to obesity. Professor Walsh and his colleagues at the Boston University School of Medicine's Whitaker Cardiovascular Institute wanted to determine whether they harmed our metabolism in any way and, specifically, if they downgraded the functioning of good fat.

To do this they fed mice a high-fat, high-sugar diet – much

like the average food intake in the Western world – and allowed them to eat as much of it as they liked. For the mice, it was like being at a twenty-four-hour 'all you can eat' buffet. They revelled in it, nibbling away at what they fancied whenever they felt like it. After eight weeks it was crunch time. The mice were weighed and tested to see what changes, if any, had taken place in their bodies. In fact, the transformations were remarkable, though not in a good way.

Not only had the animals gained weight and unhealthy white body fat, but they had become insulin resistant, losing the ability to control blood sugar and greatly increasing the risk of diabetes. This could have been predicted. But what was less expected was the impact on good fat, which seemed to flounder under the influence of the average Western diet. Too much fat and sugar had totally confused the metabolism of the mice, leaving their good fat engorged with lipids and unable to burn calories in the way it should.

What was going on? Professor Walsh and his team teased apart the facts and figures from their study. Gorging on fat and sugar had caused cells in the bodies of the mice to dysfunction. As a result, the good fat cells were deprived of the oxygen they needed to fire up the powerhouse mitochondria within them. They started to shrivel and die. Unable to produce heat and burn fatty acids, the good brown fat cells piled up with lipids and oils. They were effectively turning white and beginning to resemble the very body fat they were designed to blast away.

It adds to the convincing case for changing our diets

for the better. Too much sugar and fat settles as the kind of body fat we need to avoid; reducing our intake of these pariahs could allow our good fat to thrive.

Meal Scheduling

Our ancestors not only ate less of the bad stuff, they consumed food more sparingly. It seems sensible to suggest that were we to replicate that behaviour, if only occasionally, then it would not do our good fat any harm. It might even trigger it into the kind of heightened activity that kept our ancestors slender millenia ago.

It's this thinking that got researchers wondering if intermittent fasting – an approach that has gained in popularity as a means to weight loss following studies that showed moderate food restriction can have hugely beneficial effects on obesity and on health – could potentially boost good fat in the process.

Sporadic studies on animals over the years have suggested that mini-fasting episodes can indeed have a positive effect on the calorie-burning powers of good fat. It is far from scientific confirmation, but a spate of newer findings are adding fuel to the metabolic fire. What seems to be important is meal scheduling: that is, timetabling in chunks of time in a day when food is not consumed. This approach – which is incredibly easy to adopt – will form the basis of the Ice Diet eating plans that follow in Part Two of the book.

To demonstrate the effects it can have, let's look at some of the recent studies. A group of biologists at the

Salk Institute found that when mice on a high-fat diet were restricted to eating for eight hours a day, they consumed just as much as those who were allowed to eat around the clock.[14] But after 100 days, the differences between the two groups of animals were astonishing. Mice that had nibbled throughout the day, repeatedly snacking just because they could, became obese even though they had consumed the same total amount of calories as the group of animals forced to 'fast' for sixteen hours.

The nosh-around-the-clock mice had raised blood sugar levels, fatty livers and other metabolic ills. By wrapping up eating into eight hours, fasting offered protection against these and obesity. Crucially, it also revved up the body's stores of good fat, which became more active when food was not in constant supply. Others have hinted that short-term fasts are beneficial in similar ways. When exposed to cool temperatures, good fat cells suck up more glucose from the bloodstream if fasting has taken place beforehand.[15]

Of course, there are caveats to the existing studies. They have been carried out on mice, for starters, animals that are not exposed to the twenty-four-hour opening times of fast-food joints and supermarkets. And their body clocks are different. In the Salk Institute research, the mice ate at night, when they were most active. There's no guarantee that the results could be replicated in humans, though the scientists are optimistic.

However, there are clear signs that the health consequences of a poor diet are not just down to *what* we eat, but *when* we eat it. Meal scheduling has been shown to help people lose weight and to do so without triggering hunger pangs and the gnawing emptiness that comes with most calorie-restrictive diets. It's an approach that I have adopted with relative ease and find it slots effortlessly into my cool-living lifestyle. The way we live now has evolved to create a mismatch between our body clocks and our eating schedules. And it's one of the best methods we have of recalibrating our systems.

Fruit and Veg

A surprising discovery, even for the scientists who made it, is that a natural compound found in many fruit and vegetables seems to switch on good fat. Ursolic acid, the richest food source of which is apples and in particular the peel on the outside of the fruit, is also found in basil, bilberries, cranberries, elderflower, peppermint, rosemary, lavender, oregano, thyme and prunes. It had already been shown to be helpful for people who had gained weight by boosting the action of a protein that helps sugars to be removed from the bloodstream. But a trial on obese rats[16] found it to be even more powerful than was expected. For six weeks, the fat mice were given a high-fat diet and allowed to eat as much of the food as they wanted. They were split into three groups: one had just the food, while the others were supplemented with either 0.27g or 0.14g of ursolic acid per 100g of the food provided. This is a lot more than we'd normally get from food on a daily basis. To put things into perspective, an apple with peel provides around 0.05g of ursolic acid.

Apart from this, the lifestyles of the mice were pretty similar throughout the test. They did the same amount of activity, for example. But when the researchers came to analyse their findings, the results differed hugely between the groups. The mice on the ursolic-supplemented diet ate more than their counterparts but lost weight and gained lean muscle tissue. Experts were unsure how or why, but the addition of the supplement also triggered an increase in good fat.

The benefits combined were good news. Because ursolic acid increased the amount of skeletal muscle, the animals' strength and endurance levels increased so that, in principle, they could exercise harder for longer. With more muscle tissue and greater good fat activity, their capacity for burning calories also soared. Indeed, the researchers showed that ursolic acid-fed mice burned more calories than mice that didn't get the supplement.

As yet, we don't know how well humans absorb larger intakes of ursolic acid, but the findings provide food for thought. Including ursolic-rich foods in the diet will certainly do no harm as they are nutrient-packed and also provide valuable fibre. And it could be a step towards better brown fat behaviour.

Peppers

Igniting your taste buds with certain hot peppers is another proven way to boost good fat and up your calorie burn. Peppers contain a group of chemicals called capsaicinoids that have been shown to have powerful effects on both metabolism and the amount of food we eat. Daily consumption of just 2mg of capsaicinoids before meals led to people selecting food containing 74 fewer calories.[17]

Within the fiery compounds, it is an active ingredient called capsaicin that is among the most potent. And the hotter the peppers you eat, the more of it you get. Chilli peppers, for example, are among the richest sources of capsaicin with 2mg of it found in just 75g of chopped-up chillis. Trials on mice have shown that capsaicinoids raise metabolism and elevate good fat activity. Could it have the same effect on humans too?

To find out, a group of Japanese researchers added chilli powder to a variety of high-fat and high-protein meals given to a group of female volunteers at breakfast time.[18] Each woman ate the same ratio of foods containing the same amount of calories. Some of the meals contained added red pepper, others were served without. Although the participants preferred the taste of the less-spicy food first thing in the morning, the chilli-spiced meals resulted in enhanced energy expenditure and calorie burn by the body after they had been consumed.

It proved intriguing enough for the researchers to decide to delve more deeply into the chilli effect with further studies.[19, 20, 21] One involving eighteen healthy young men required the subjects to place their feet on blocks of ice intermittently while PET scans detected levels of good fat. Ten of them were shown to have active good fat, eight had none that was visible. Next, things got interesting. Both groups were given capsules of capsaicinoids (and not the spiciest variety), as well as a placebo capsule, to see how their bodies responded.

In the good fat group, calorie burning increased after the pepper pills but not after the placebo. There were no changes in calorie-burn among the other men. Let's be clear that we are not talking colossal increases in metabolism here. After ingesting the hot peppers, the good fat group experienced a calorie-burn rise of about 4 calories an hour, which would result in a very modest weight loss over time.

But the findings do open the floodgates for more research. Scientists are particularly interested in finding a cocktail of ingredients, including capsaicinoids, that might serve to trick the brain into thinking it is being cooled and coax good fat into gobbling up more calories than usual. Caffeine might be one such ingredient. An early study[22] showed how adding 3g of red pepper and 200mg of caffeine in the form of a cup of coffee taken with a meal caused an increase in energy burned and a decrease in food consumed. Green tea, also thought to trigger metabolism, could also be added to the mix. It raises the question of whether the future could see a chilli pepper-based pill being popped to boost good fat on a daily basis.

Other Foods

Many other foods are just beginning to catch the interest of scientists when it comes to their ability to trigger the kind of changes that lead to more calories being burned.

One such food group is dairy. Using thermal imaging, Professor Michael Symonds has shown that drinking milk results in a 0.7 °C rise in good fat temperature, suggesting it is spurred into greater levels of activity.[23] When others have looked at the thermogenic effects of different foods, they've also found that while protein boosts the metabolic response, too much fat has no benefit.[24, 25] Some fascinating thermal images taken before and after a 13-year-old ate a breakfast of porridge made with 25g of oats, 70ml full-fat milk and brown sugar showed clearly how good fat temperature was increased five minutes after eating.[26]

So far, no food has been proven to be a magical good fat booster. How good fat responds to different food groups is a new and emerging scientific topic, but is beginning to captivate researchers in their hordes. There's a real possibility that their findings could eventually enable food manufacturers to include a new category of health advice on food packaging. Professor Symonds told me that 'potentially we could add a thermogenic index to food labels to show whether that product would increase or decrease heat production within brown fat'. In other words, it is feasible that we could check on labels whether a food would speed up or slow down the amount of calories we burn via its ability to fire good fat into motion.

Drugs

Wouldn't it be more convenient to take a drug that boosts good fat activity? We all like an easy option and a pill you can pop for weight loss is the most elusive of all types of medication. Unsurprisingly, the concept that we might be able to treat fat with fat is intriguing to pharmaceutical companies who, realizing its marketing and results potential, have embarked on a race to find a pill or injectible that could stimulate good fat without having to make any changes to your diet or lifestyle.

No doubt dazzled by pound signs – it's been estimated that the pay-off for a good fat booster would be huge, somewhere in the region of £15 billion pounds annually – they foresee a future in which we might be able to go for fat jabs in the same way people visit a surgery to erase wrinkles with a syringe and a needle. There would be medical advantages to such a treatment, of course. If the obesity epidemic could be 'treated' in this way, then the risk of death from diseases associated with excessive fatness would come tumbling down. But is it really possible to get a shot of good fat that would prevent us having to make any effort at all with our diets and lifestyle?

Thyroid replacement therapy is known to drive good fat formation, but brings unwanted side effects so is a no-go. Another ingredient found in over-the-counter decongestant medicines for coughs and cold, called ephedrine, was thought to be a possibility. Could it activate good fat without having to expose yourself to the cold, experts wondered? The idea stemmed from earlier research suggesting that ephedrine seemed to cause weight loss by stimulating a release of the messenger molecule norepinephrine, increasing the number of calories burned. Since brown adipose tissue has receptors for norepinephrine, other researchers reasoned the drug would spur it into activity.

It turns out to be not that simple. While ephedrine does help with weight loss, it's not clear if and how it uses good fat to do so. Taking an ephedrine solution has been shown, for instance, to have more of an effect on good fat-boosting in lean people than obese.[27] Others have questioned whether it works at all. In one trial,[28] a group of ten subjects were given a jab of either ephedrine or a saline solution, and after each injection were asked to wear cooling vests that chilled their bodies to 57 °C for two hours. Measurements of good fat were taken after each cooling episode using PET-CT scans.

What did they show? Good fat activity was similar after both jabs; the injections and the cooling vests burned the same total amounts of calories. But there was a crucial difference. After wearing the ice vests for a couple of hours, good fat activity was sent soaring. Cool temperatures once again reigned supreme, with the researchers at the Joslin Diabetes Center concluding that getting people to wear the cooling vests to help them to lose weight might be an option.

Drug companies are not stopping there. Huge pharma companies including Genotech, backed by Roche, and Eli Lilly have looked at a hormone called fibroblast growth factor 21 (FGF21), known to boost good fat. Other potential pills are in the pipeline. Cambridge University scientists found a protein called BMP8B, made in the brain and in good fat itself, which turns up the body's thermostat to stimulate good fat to burn calories.[29] It could be that a drug is developed to target the pathway that fires the protein into action. Targeting irisin, the hormone produced by muscles that helps to brown white fat after exercise, is another possibility.

I'm in no doubt that, at some point in the future, there will be a drug available that promises to spur brown fat into action and help to combat obesity. Natural ways to enhance our body's ability to ward off flab, though, remain the most effective solution and the beauty of the Ice Diet is that it is cheap, easy to do and has no nasty side effects.

Good Fat and Your Health

If you follow the Ice Diet programme, designed to maximize your fat-burning potential, then you will lose weight in a steady way and trick your body into burning more calories than it is at the moment. You will almost certainly become leaner and more toned, especially if you add the exercise programme included later in the book. But is there any evidence that good fat can do more than that? Recent experiments have indeed revealed that good fat's benefits go far beyond calorie burning. They have been linked to preventing diseases of ageing and some of the biggest killers of our generation:

Osteoporosis and Bone-Thinning

There's an intriguing relationship between good fat and bone density. Clifford Rosen, Professor of Medicine at Tufts University School of Medicine in Boston, is studying mice that cannot make good fat and was astonished by the state of their bones. When exposed to cold temperatures, the mice without brown fat quickly lose bone density. 'The animals have the worst bone density we have ever seen,' he told the *New York Times*.[30] 'I see osteoporotic bones all the time, but, oh my God, these are the extreme.' It's a complex interplay and while Professor Rosen and other researchers know that good fat somehow protects bone strength, they are not yet sure how or why this happens.[31]

Type 2 Diabetes

People with higher levels of good fat in their bodies have been shown to have better blood sugar control, high insulin sensitivity and an inner weapon to fight diabetes.[32] Researchers at the Joslin Diabetes Center were the first to discover how good fat works by hoovering up sugars from the blood, improving the body's insulin control[33] and helping to reduce the risk for Type 2 diabetes. Now it's known that the effect is heightened when people are exposed to cool temperatures.

For people of South Asian origin, who have long been known to have a higher risk of diabetes, it could even be a lack of good fat that is partly to blame. When Dutch researchers analysed a group of healthy 25-year-old South Asian men and a similar group of Caucasians, they found the volume of metabolically active good fat to be more than one-third lower in the Asian group. Interestingly, the

South Asian men also shivered sooner when exposed to cold temperatures, suggesting that it was recruited to keep them warm with so little good fat present.[34]

Heart Disease

For healthy people there is little doubt that cooler living can help shape leaner and healthier bodies by activating brown fat cells and burning off excess fat. That, in turn, also accelerates the removal of triglycerides, or lipids, from the bloodstream – precisely the kind of fatty molecules that, when they are present in excess, are known to raise the risk of metabolic syndrome, a cluster of symptoms that can increase the chance of getting conditions like diabetes, strokes and heart disease.

However, the cold is something of a double-edged sword when it comes to heart protection. In people who already have heart disease and hardening of the arteries, exposure to the cold might not be such a good thing. Not because the shock of cold temperatures could prove too much for them, but because some small studies have hinted that activation of good fat might cause higher levels of 'bad' LDL cholesterol in their bloodstream.[35] It's one of the reasons why it's imperative to have a check-up before attempting any of the strategies in the Ice Diet.

Why Good Fat Is So Good

It's astounding to think that such a recent rediscovery could have such a dramatic impact on our health. Initially, when I found out about how I could activate good fat in my own body, I'll admit the attraction was just about the extra calories that could be burned, the weight that could be shed. However, the more I have learned about its capacity to enhance our health, the more inspired I've become. There are heaps of benefits, as we've seen in this chapter, and the list keeps on growing. But here's what we know, so far, on why good fat is so good:

- It gobbles up calories and helps us lose weight.
- It sucks sugars from the bloodstream, protecting against the threat of diabetes.
- It hoovers up blood fats, lowering the risk of metabolic disorders and heart disease in healthy people.
- In different ways it responds to cool living, exercise and healthy foods, all of which are the underpinnings of a healthy lifestyle.
- Boosting good fat can fight diseases of ageing: we might live longer.

3 The Ice Edge

What I've found as I've delved deeper into the world of cool science is that people have wildly varying theories about how ice can help us to lose weight and stay healthy. Some of these ideas are highly convincing and are already backed by volumes of research, others are less credible. Knowing how quickly scientific viewpoints can change, especially in the field of good fat, ice and metabolism, I'm loathe to dismiss some of this fringe science altogether. It's left field, certainly, but much of it is work presented by medical professionals I've encountered who have no reason to mislead the public.

In sport and exercise science, the study of 'marginal gains' is considered key in the success of Olympic athletes. It was the visionary and highly successful former British Cycling coach, Dave Brailsford, who first brought to prominence the idea that by breaking down and identifying every tiny aspect of an athlete's performance and then making just a 1 per cent improvement in each area, the athlete's overall performance can be significantly enhanced. Before the London 2012 Olympics, Brailsford and his scientific support team got cyclists to spend hours in wind tunnels to find the optimal riding posture. They wore one-piece skin suits to reduce drag. They took their own pillows and bedding when they travelled to events to minimize the risk of illness and poor sleep.

The micro-improvements could never be hugely significant on their own. But as part of an overall approach, they are far from trivial factors. It's the aggregation of these sorts of marginal gains that can provide physical and physiological improvements. It certainly worked for the cyclists. The British team had their most successful Olympic Games ever when they adopted the 'no stone unturned' approach.

And that, I think, is how we should view some of the theories outlined in this chapter. They are fledgling concepts, untried and untested in the eyes of the wider scientific community. They might be the seed of something bigger or they might not be. Individually, they are unlikely to make a huge difference to calorie burning. But when these approaches are added in fine veneers to the rock-solid principles behind the Ice Diet, they could possibly have an impact. They are an Ice Dieter's tools for marginal gains. I've included them because I believe them to be important in the overall movement towards cooler living. But also because dieting and weight loss are prone to drudgery and these bring a fun element to the whole battle of the bulge.

Negative Ice Calories (icals)

One of the most agreeable new ice theories is being put forward by Dr Brian Weiner, a New Jersey-based gastro-enterologist, who told me about a discovery that helped him reduce his own middle-aged paunch. Dr Weiner said the pounds had crept on around his tummy and enough was enough, it was time to do something about it before the slippery slope became irreversible.

In a ruthless examination of his diet he decided that the first thing to change was his regular ice-cream habit. He loved the creamiest, most calorific varieties, he said, and so switched them for non-dairy, ice-based sorbets and crushed ice drinks. 'Within weeks of doing that and increasing my exercise, I lost weight,' Dr Weiner reported. 'And I really believe that the added ice was playing a role.'

When ice is eaten, the brain signals for the body to heat up the cold, alien substance. By the time ice reaches the stomach it is close to body temperature. That process requires energy. Quite how much energy has yet to be substantiated, but Weiner has made his own calculations and estimates it works out at 5 calories per 25g of ice. 'I sat looking at the nutritional labels on the ice desserts I had started eating and it suddenly struck me that it was all wrong,' Weiner said. 'They were listed as containing 100 calories, but that didn't take into account the energy required by the body to melt the ice for digestion. When you deducted that, the calorific total was more like 72 per serving.'

Going by Weiner's ical theories, were you to ingest one litre of ice daily – easier than you think if you take an ice lolly and a low-sugar slush puppie or fruit-based frappuccino – you could burn about 160 calories, the energy equivalent of a yoga session or power walking a mile. 'It doesn't sound much, but over a year that equates to an overall loss of 10–12 pounds,' he said. 'It is in line with what health authorities recommend we should aim to lose.'

Weiner argues that ice-containing foods and anything eaten when partially or wholly frozen should be measured in icals, a term for the figure reached when the extra calories used to bring ice to body temperature is deducted. In 2010 he submitted the story of his own ice-munching habits and his hunch about icals to the editors of the widely read medical journal *Annals of Internal Medicine*, who proceeded to published it.[1] 'I'm not suggesting that people consume only ice and ice-based products, but that some ice consumption is a highly effective adjunct to exercise and a healthy diet,' Dr Weiner told me.

He's not the only medical expert to be intrigued by the weight loss potential of ice. At the University of Nottingham's Queen's Medical Centre, Professor Symonds is looking at the ways ice creams and lollies might boost metabolism by activating good body fat. Healthy female volunteers aged 18–35 are asked to arrive at the Nottingham labs before breakfast so that they are in a fasted state and to change into a light cotton vest and shorts. Professor Symonds and researcher James Law then measure their skin temperature and heart rate and take baseline thermal image readings using their high-tech cameras for 10–20 minutes.

Then the subjects are given a food stimulus in the form

of a bowl of ice cream, an ice-cold glass of water, a glass of room temperature water or a sweetened milk drink. The team then continues to track 'thermal imaging responses' in the neck area for up to 2 hours after the cold and room temperature drinks are consumed. Early results are promising. When the ice cream is eaten, there is an immediate drop in temperature in the neck area where good brown fat is stored, suggesting that cold desserts can trigger activity, albeit fairly briefly. During the hour after eating the ice cream, body temperature rises steadily and is back to the baseline level shortly after that. Although the researchers stress that more work needs to be done to confirm the effect, it could be that cold foods and drinks are indeed a veritable weight-loss aid.

In the meantime, Dr Weiner still aims to consume one litre of ice a day to keep his weight down. He avoids ice cubes which, he says, can damage the enamel of the teeth, and has invested in a margarita maker in which he crushes ice. And he still eats his ice-based sorbets instead of ice cream.

How icals Are Calculated

Dr Weiner's ical calculation is based on the energy it takes for the body to warm and melt ice as it is being consumed. By his estimation, if you were to eat a litre of ice, the metabolic energy needed to bring it from freezer temperature (-20 °C) to freezing point at 0 °C is around 20 calories. There is then a considerable amount of metabolic energy required to melt ice from its solid state at 0 °C to liquid – an additional cost of 80 calories. To bring it to room temperature, another 37 calories per litre is required. Taking into account the fact that the metabolism varies, Dr Weiner has estimated that, in total, about 160 calories are burned in melting and bringing one litre of ice from the freezer to body temperature. That amounts to about 5 calories per 25g of ice consumed.

Using this theory, it is interesting to work out how many calories you might be 'saving' by eating icy foods, bearing in mind that a pure ice product requires energy to melt the ice to body temperature so the calorie count is likely to be less than that listed. Below are a few examples of how labels might change if the ical theory were to be adopted. It's all a bit of fun, but provides (cool) food for thought in the process.

Calories Per Average Serving
(ical values are approximate)

Crushed plain ice (500ml): 0 calories (minus 80 icals)

R Whites Lemonade Lolly (75ml): 60 calories (42 icals)

Del Monte Fresh Juice Lolly (75ml): 61 calories (43 icals)

Slush Puppie Classic (per 100ml): 37.6 calories (32 icals)

Jubbly Strawberry Lolly (62ml): 16 calories (14 icals)

Starbucks Grande Mango Passion Fruit Frappuccino (473ml): 192 calories (170 icals)

Classic Margarita (200ml): 145 calories (105 icals)

Mr Freeze ice pops (20ml): 5 calories (0 icals)
Tesco Goodness Rocket Lollies (58ml): 43 calories
   (33 icals)
Lemon sorbet (100g): 122 calories (83 icals)
Mr Bubble ice lolly (74ml): 51 calories (36 icals)
Calippo Orange (105ml): 100 calories (72 icals)

When Is a Calorie Not a Calorie?

The negative calorie theory is not as far-fetched as it sounds. One of the long-standing truisms of dieting is that a calorie is a calorie; that the more of them we consume (and the less we expend), the fatter we will get. But what if everything we thought we knew about calories was wrong? Several studies in recent years have thrown open the debate about how calories are calculated, questioning conventional wisdom about which foods are really slowing down weight loss. Their conclusion? Not only are many of the calorie contents listed on food labels and in diet books inaccurate, the calories from certain foods affect the body in different ways.

How Are Calories Calculated?

Existing calorie tables were first put together more than a hundred years ago by an agricultural chemist called Wilbur Olin Atwater. Using a device called a 'bomb calorimeter', Atwater literally burned samples of food and then measured the amount of energy released from the heat this produced. He worked out that every gram of carbohydrates produced 4 calories, every gram of fat produced 9 calories and every gram of protein produced 4 calories. What concerns experts now is that Atwater's figures are estimates based on averages that don't take into account variations in food make-up, preparation methods and processing techniques.

Why Lightly Cooked Food is Better

There is plenty of evidence that cooking alters the structure of food by softening it and making it easier and less time-consuming for our bodies to digest. It can make food more palatable and enjoyable, but will also reduce the effort required to eat it. In many cases, when it comes to calorie ingestion, the less processed it is (that means minimal bashing, chopping, heating and cooking), the better.

That was what Rachel Carmody, a researcher at Harvard University's Department of Human Evolutionary Biology, found when she examined the effects of two forms of food preparation on the calories available in the same food. Previously, Carmody had shown that sweet potatoes contain more calories when they are cooked because the starch they contain can be better digested by the body. But in her latest study the scientist looked at whether the preparation of lean organic beef had any effect on calories ingested. She compared cooked and raw minced beef to see if the calorie content differed when fed to laboratory mice.

What she found was that, unsurprisingly, cooked meat was easy to digest and that the mice lost 2g of body weight on raw meat but just 1g on a cooked meat diet. The findings took into account their normal diets so were independent of that. By cooking the meat, proteins were broken down so that they were easier to digest. It could also be that heat kills bacteria, meaning the immune system has less work to do when food is cooked, another energy saving for the body. It means that raw or lightly steamed vegetables, lightly cooked fish and medium to rare cooked red meat could have fewer calories per plateful than overcooked food.

Ice-cold Water for Weight Loss – Really?

Jennifer Lopez is among the many celebrities who has said she drinks ice-cold water to boost her metabolism. Can this really work? A decade ago a published study[2] suggested that drinking 500ml of ice-cold water (22 °C) increased metabolism by 30 per cent compared to baseline, while drinking water at 37 °C produced a smaller increase in metabolism. This effect was evident within 10 minutes, peaked at 30–40 minutes, and lasted over 1 hour. This study, however, was the only one that demonstrated such a positive effect of water on metabolism.

Then, in 2006, another group of researchers challenged this assertion with a study of their own[3] after several similar studies cited that cold water had no effect on metabolism. This team used a more accurate form of indirect calorimetry and gave distilled water to eliminate the possibility of an ionic effect on metabolism. Their study did indeed demonstrate an increase in metabolism after drinking cold water, but it was minimal. That change was likely due to the energy required by the body to bring the water to its internal temperature in a similar mechanism to the 'icals' theory.

Is cold water of any benefit in weight loss? Not significantly when it comes to metabolism and good fat. What it provides is a sense of fullness, and thirst may be misinterpreted as hunger that really just requires a drink of water rather than a snack. Don't stop drinking cold water, but don't count on it to be your magic bullet for weight loss.

But an icy drink might make your workout last longer . . .

A pre-workout ice ingestion could help you to work harder for longer, burning extra calories in the process. In warm weather or hot environments like gyms and yoga studios, the body diverts blood away from the muscles to the skin for cooling. That's partly why exercise often feels harder in hotter weather, why you struggle to keep going for as long as usual. Exercise physiologists suspect many people quit a workout more readily when it's hot either because their muscles are starved of blood or because the heart eventually struggles to beat fast enough to satisfy all the demands for blood.

But a study by New Zealand researchers in the journal *Medicine and Science in Sports and Exercise* showed how slushy ice drinks help to prevent these adverse side effects.[4] Crushed ice had previously been shown to lower brain temperature in lab animals better than cold water; when sugary solutions are mixed in they become even colder than plain ice cubes, which is why the New Zealand scientists opted for slushy drinks in the experiment.

In the trial, male athletes were given a syrup-flavoured ice slush just before running on a treadmill in a hot room and were able to keep going for an average of 50 minutes before they had to stop. When they drank only syrup-flavoured cold water they could run for an average of 40 minutes. It seems the ice drink probably lowered their body temperature before they ran, letting them keep going longer before their bodies became too hot. The slushy ice approach is also being tested at the University of Montana's Center for Work Physiology and Exercise Metabolism and could, quite feasibly, become common practice prior to hot sports competitions.

If you're not a fan of slushy drinks, plain cold water could have a boosting effect too. A group of cyclists taking part in another study drank 300ml of either a cold (4 °C) or a warm (37 °C) drink during 30 minutes of pedalling. They were also asked to consume 100ml of the same drink every 10 minutes during exercise while sport scientists at Loughborough University monitored their rectal and skin temperatures, heart rate and sweat rate.[5] They found that what they called 'the heat-reduced physiological strain' that came with drinking the cold drink significantly boosted endurance capacity by as much as 6 per cent. In other words, the cyclists could keep pedalling for longer before having to stop through sweaty exhaustion.

But be careful when you drink: preliminary evidence suggests sipping ice-cold drinks post exercise, when you probably think you most need them after working up a sweat, might not be such a good thing. A hard workout also triggers good fat into calorie-burning mode and taking ice immediately afterwards could counteract that. There are other disadvantages. After running or a gym session the body uses energy to dissipate the excess heat that builds up during exercise. If you ingest large amounts of ice-cold products following exercise, then some of the heat that was generated by the workout would be neutralized by the coolness of the ice. Ultimately, that would reduce some of the long-term calorie-burning benefits of exercise.

Ice Chambers

I first came across the use of ice as a fitness-boosting recovery aid over a decade ago when I was commissioned to interview the then England rugby players Lawrence Dallaglio and Joe Worsley who, at the time, were making regular trips to an Olympic training centre in Poland for a treatment that involved them standing in a cryotherapy chamber – essentially a deep freeze for human beings – at temperatures that the body can barely withstand.

It seemed ludicrous at the time. Why would anyone want to put themselves through a 'therapy' that was a kind of torture? I was told that liquid nitrogen was used to cool the air inside the sealed cryotherapy unit to -135 °C (-211 °F) – to put that into perspective, many ski resorts are forced to close when weather conditions drop to a potentially dangerous -35 °C. *Brrr.*

Now, though, everyone is at it. Formula One racing drivers, athletes, footballers, actresses – Demi Moore visits a cryotherapy chamber to keep her youthful looks – and even James Bond in the form of actor Daniel Craig are said to have used whole-body ice chambers to get into shape. Double Olympic champion Mo Farah has used the cryotherapy approach, claiming it helps him to recover so that he is ready for another training session. 'You work hard, it's important to recover as quick as you can . . . It really helps to recover when you've done hard training or racing,' he has been quoted as saying. Red Bull Formula One driver Mark Webber has credited chilling out in cryogenic chambers at temperatures of -130 °C with aiding his performance.

You can find cryotherapy ice chambers at fashionable health spas and at stand-alone, walk-in clinics. Mobile units are ferried to international sporting events. As I write, athletes at the European Athletics Championships are linking cryotherapy visits with helping them to win gold medals. Even I have been tempted to give it a go to see what all the fuss is about. So what's it like?

Each session in the chamber began with a 30-second 'acclimatization' blast of air cooled to -57 °C. Temperatures then plummeted dramatically and, after being frozen at -80 °C to -135 °C, as the rugby players and footballers would do, I emerged to complete 20 minutes of cardiovascular exercise on a treadmill, rowing machine or stationary bike positioned just outside the chamber.

With athletes, the whole procedure is sometimes repeated twice a day after each training session. My therapist at a plush spa with ice chambers told me how crucial it is to keep your extremities covered and to wear goggles or a specially designed mask, 'otherwise your eyeballs might freeze'. It's not what you might call a pleasurable or relaxing experience. I could stand only just over a minute in the deep-freeze environment. But the benefits seem to be worth it for those who persist with it regularly. According to sports medicine experts, it accelerates the body's recovery process to five times quicker than normal, which allows for a greater intensity and a higher volume of training. It improves blood flow and gets rid of waste products such as lactic acid that can limit performance. One leading Premier League rugby coach told me his players could generally achieve two weeks' worth of training in one week when they are using cryotherapy.

There are other purported advantages too, such as a raised production of enzymes and hormones, including testosterone, which helps you to bounce back not only from sport and exercise, but illness. In my view, it all comes back to marginal gains. Cryotherapy is not a magic cure by any means. But it is developing a huge following among those who feel it can enhance an otherwise healthy lifestyle with plenty of exercise and a good diet.

Ice Vests

To footballers, athletes and others who are required to play sport in searing heat, this unlikely item of clothing provides a welcome alternative to a warm-up. Cooling 'ice' jackets are widely used to bring down the body temperature before top-level sports competitions that take place in hot environments. Team GB used them during the Beijing 2008 Olympics and Adidas provided Spanish, German and Argentinian footballers with pre-cooling vests and sleeves before the 2014 World Cup in Brazil.

Designed so that there is no ice in direct contact with the skin, the garments are made to be stored in a freezer to maintain a temperature of close to freezing for 15–20 minutes, allowing players a suitable cooling period before playing in heat of 25 °C or above. They are undoubtedly helpful in sport. But could the high-tech cooling vest have a wider role to play for the rest of us?

Evidence that they could be useful for weight loss came in the form of a study carried out by Dr Aaron Cypess and his team at the Joslin Diabetes Center. It was the same trial that was looking to see if the drug ephedrine could be used to activate good fat on cue. Volunteers were given injections of either the drug or a saline solution and were also asked to wear the special cooling vests with water pumped into them at 13 °C. Fat activity was then measured. While they concluded that the drug didn't work any better than the saline solution, when the cooling vests were worn for two hours they stimulated good fat significantly.[6]

Wearing a cooling vest is not the most desirable way to send your good fat roaring, but neither is it particularly unpleasant. I've tried it and, after a few minutes of discomfort, the coolness becomes tolerable. You almost forget you are wearing an ice gilet. Along with Adidas, other companies now market cooling vests for general use. One of them, Hyperwear, manufactures gel-filled vests and is developing a patented brown-fat cooling vest called CoolBurn for further research studies, designed to stimulate brown adipose tissue to fight obesity and diabetes. They aren't cheap (expect to pay around £100), but if you are serious about cooling, then they may be worth a try.

Ice Gloves

The concept of an ice glove was something of a revelation to me when I first heard about it from Paul Strzelecki, a professor at the University of Manchester. Paul had been working with researchers at Stanford University who had developed a glove that they claimed could rapidly cool all-over body temperature and enhance exercise recovery as well as helping to explain why muscles get tired. They claim the device is so effective for sports people that it could give a boost 'better than steroids . . . and it's not illegal'.

What intrigued me was the idea of wearing something on the hand. It seemed an unlikely place for body cooling. Yet for more than a decade, Stamford biologists Professor Craig Heller and Dennis Grahn have been researching how best to cool the body and have found that specialized heat-transfer veins in the palms of the hands are key. It was a discovery they made by studying black bears – animals that, with a thick coat of fur and a layer of subcutaneous fat, are extremely well-insulated. It's necessary during winter, but what happened when spring hit, the scientists wondered. How did the bears avoid overheating?

Their research showed that the bears, like most mammals, have in-built radiators – areas of the body that have no hair or fur and feature a network of veins called AVAs (arteriovenous anastomoses) close to the skin's surface that don't supply nutrition to the skin and vary in the amount of blood that flows to the area. On a rabbit, these are in the ears. On bears, though, they're on the pads of their feet. And humans seem to have them on the face, feet and also the palms of our hands.

By taking advantage of these veins, the pair found they could dramatically reduce athletes' core temperatures and improve performance in the process. It's a milder approach to cooling and, as such, a more practical solution than a full-body water submersion or other strategies. Yet, the Stamford duo claim, equally effective.

So, does it work? Initially it was tested on college athletes doing various types of exercise, everything from sprinting to weightlifting. In every case, recovery rates improved dramatically compared to occasions when the glove had not been used. As a result, a commercial version of the RTX (Rapid Thermal Exchange) Cooling Glove (which costs around £1,050) has been adopted by elite track and field teams, the San Francisco 49ers and Manchester United Football Club.

Its biggest test came during the 2014 World Cup in Brazil when it was used by the German football team. Players donned the gloves in the dressing room at half-time, immediately reducing their temperatures. By all accounts, the stamina of the team was remarkable. And guess what? They won the tournament.

Ice Baths

Dunking in a bathtub filled with ice water soared to popularity as a post-workout regimen when top sportsmen and women were pictured taking a chilly dip to supposedly reduce soreness, inflammation of muscles and speed up recovery after intense exercise. Everyone from the marathon world-record holder Paula Radcliffe to David Beckham has used the cringe-inducing approach, which involves spending several often painful minutes (and I know because I've tried it) in the freezing tub.

And what works for the elite generally filters down to the masses. Ice baths and plunge pools have become a popular way for gym-goers and recreational exercisers to finish a session in the belief that they are repairing their bodies more quickly for the next bout of exercise. In theory, the vastly improved recovery time means that you can perform high-intensity workouts more often and, therefore, reach your fitness goals more quickly. But does the ice-bath theory hold water?

So widespread is their use that university sports science departments are keen to determine whether there are indeed any benefits from the practice. One study[7] had twenty active young men running downhill for 40 minutes at a gradient of −10 per cent. Afterwards, half of them were asked to stand up to their thighs in a recycling bin filled with water chilled to 5 °C for a tear-inducing 20 minutes. The others were lucky – they escaped the ice-bath routine altogether.

Post-workout measurements of muscle soreness while walking downstairs, quadricep muscle strength and thigh circumference were then taken at intervals from one hour to three days. Researchers also checked the blood concentration of a substance called plasma chemokine ligand 2 (CCL2), a marker for inflammation. What did they find?

Interestingly, their results chalked up no difference in strength or perceived soreness between the ice-bath users and those who hadn't been subjected to the prolonged dip. Neither did thigh circumference, another measure of inflammation, differ between the groups. There was a slightly lower concentration of CCL2 in the ice-bath group, although it was not a significant improvement.

The upshot? Ice baths seemed not to have much of an effect. It surprised researchers, who had expected to see a more dramatic improvement, particularly in soreness levels, after the chilling. It's fair to point out that other studies have found the opposite to be the case. A review in the Cochrane Library[8] by a University of Ulster team found a post-workout ice bath reduced muscle soreness by 20 per cent. Even so, they also stated that there were no differences when the ice-water immersion was compared to other recovery methods (compression stockings, light jogging, warm baths), so confirmation that it is the most effective strategy still hangs in the balance.

From my own experience, ice baths help a little. I was certainly back to walking more easily after using one post-marathon. But I concede that many of the benefits might be in the mind. If it works for those at the very top of the game, then maybe it will work for you.

What's clear is that ice and its many applications are in the ascendency. Never has it been so hot to be cool. Some of the measures work while others are less convincing. In addition to those mentioned on these pages are cryosurgery (a method used to freeze out tumours in hospitals), Coolsculpting (a non-surgical method of freezing away fat that has FDA approval) and many more ice-based therapies. Those discussed in this chapter are optional measures that can be added to the Ice Diet way of living if you feel they might work for you. They are by no means compulsory.

With the science covered, we are now going to put the theory into practice. In Part Two I'll outline what you need to do to embrace cool living and get your metabolism firing. What should you eat, how should you exercise and what other steps can you take to ensure you get the most out of the Ice Diet?

PART TWO

4 Users' Manual

With the science behind the Ice Diet explained, it's time to put things into action. In this chapter I'll outline the basic principles of the Ice Diet – what and when you will be eating and how the diet plan will work in tandem with cooler living strategies to maximize your body's ability to burn calories. That, in turn, will accelerate weight loss and optimize your health.

By far the best news is that it is not in any way daunting. The Ice Diet is incredibly easy to adopt. There will be no counting calories, no hunger days, no cravings and no chance of missing out on vital nutrients by avoiding important food groups.

It will almost certainly require changes to your existing diet, but the foods you will be eating are so wholesome and delicious that I promise you won't miss the ingredients you cast aside at all. And in scheduling your mealtimes you will be surprised at how easily and painlessly you adjust to eating less often – and feeling better for it.

Remember that the interplay between diet and lifestyle is essential for weight loss on the Ice Diet. It's no good adopting only the cooling strategies in the following chapter and hoping to sweep away fat in an instant. A cool lifestyle is what's needed and that means eating, living and moving well.

Where We Go Wrong

Salt

For all its bad rap, sodium chloride, or salt, is an element essential for health. Every one of our cells needs it to function – it's required to regulate fluid balance and for nerves and muscles, including those in the heart, to work well. Too little salt can cause mental confusion, an inability to concentrate and, in extreme cases, the potentially fatal condition hyponatraemia, when body salts become so dilute it causes the brain to swell.

That said, hardly any of us get too little salt in our diets. Most of us get far too much. High salt diets are a major factor in raising blood pressure and thought to be linked to increasing hypertension as we age. Precisely how it has this effect is not clear, but it is thought that when salt intake is too high the kidneys struggle to pass it all into the urine and some ends up in the bloodstream. This then draws more water into the blood, increasing volume and pressure.

The long-term goal is to have adults cut salt to 6g daily, a total of around 1 teaspoon, and children even less. Although salt intakes have fallen slightly as food manufacturers have responded to pressure from health campaigners to reduce it, the average person still exceeds that with around 8.6g of salt a day. Adding salt at the dinner table accounts for only a tiny fraction (about 5 per cent) of the total salt we consume on a daily basis. Instead, most of it comes from highly processed foods and ready meals. It's hidden in the most unlikely places: breakfast cereals and desserts can contain more salt than a bag of crisps.

On the Ice Diet, highly processed foods and ready meals are replaced with freshly prepared, easy-to-make meals that will lower your salt intake and boost your health without making any extra effort.

Sugar

For years we thought of sugar as a natural source of energy, the kind of carbohydrate that was used by athletes to fuel their bodies. We could do worse than satisfy our sweet tooth once in a while – or could we? In recent years, studies have revealed that we had sugar all wrong. Now, there are stark warnings about the effects of sugar overload on our health. And you've already seen that one researcher has blamed it for triggering a 'death spiral' for good fat.

When sugar and sugary foods are eaten, the response is a sharp rise in levels of glucose (sugar) in the bloodstream, which forces the pancreas to pump out insulin, the hormone needed to keep blood sugar levels under control. Insulin's job is to extract glucose from the bloodstream, convert it into glycogen and store it in the liver or muscles; however, since the body has only a limited storage capacity for glycogen, excess glucose from sugars and refined carbs is then stacked away as fat, eventually causing related health issues.

One report published in *Circulation*, the journal of the

American Heart Association (AHA), linked a high intake of the sweet stuff not only to obesity but to everything from raised blood pressure to heart disease and strokes.[1] It is known to cause dental problems and is linked to diabetes[2] and metabolic disorders. It has even been linked to cancer as well as a number of other illnesses.

There's little doubt that we need to cut down. Since the 1980s, sugar consumption in the UK has increased by almost one-third to around 550g (1¼lb) per person per week, an amount that exceeds the healthy guidelines by a huge margin. Some people now get almost one-fifth of their calories from sugar. The World Health Organization (WHO) issued new guidelines suggesting that cutting sugar intake to 5 per cent of total calories would be beneficial. That's about 25g (around six teaspoons) for an adult of normal weight every day.

With fewer of us adding sugar to our tea and coffee, how are we amassing these individual sugar mountains? The answer is largely via the hidden sugars in the food we buy. It is easy to see how upper limits are reached when you consider that a single can of fizzy drink can contain 9 teaspoons of sugar and an organic, tomato-based pasta sauce has 2 teaspoons per serving.

It's not just sucrose, or table sugar, that we need to look out for – our food is increasingly sweetened with sugar forms we barely recognize. Sugars come from cane, beet or corn. Virtually anything ending in the letters 'ose' is likely to be a sugar. Of particular concern are new forms of high-calorie sweeteners that are cheaply made and widely used, such as high-fructose corn syrup or HFCS.

Sweetness in the Ice Diet will be limited and will come mostly in the form of natural sugars that are not as harmful to health.

Refined Carbs

Consumption of refined carbohydrates, such as white bread, white pasta and rice, as well as cakes, biscuits and snacks, is now so high that they are considered a prime reason why so many people are overweight.

Like sugar, too many refined carbohydrates cause the blood sugar (glucose) to rise sharply and the pancreas to pump out insulin ferociously to extract it from the bloodstream, convert it to glycogen and store it in the liver or muscles. Over time, this process is compromised. About an hour and a half after eating refined carbs you feel hungry again, so you eat more and the result is that since the body has a limited capacity for glycogen storage, excess is stored as body fat.

Eventually, overloaded by the sugary demands, the body becomes 'insulin resistant' and this paves the way for Type 2 diabetes. Since insulin is the main hormone responsible for depositing fat cells, many obesity experts now propose that a lower and healthier carbohydrate diet will reduce insulin levels and release stored body fat for use as fuel.

Spikes in blood sugar levels from eating too many refined carbs are now linked to a host of other unhealthy side effects. They are known to have an effect on the action of the hormone leptin, secreted by fat cells to act on a part of the brain that suppresses appetite and controls metabolism. When someone gains weight, leptin levels rise in a bid to maintain the equilibrium. But huge swings in blood sugar can lead to 'leptin resistance', meaning the hormone is unable to do its job and the body settles at a weight often far from its optimum for health.

The crucial message is that not all carbs need to be avoided. But it is certainly advisable to steer clear of sugar and refined carbohydrates, and those foods with a high glycaemic index (GI) as explained below, as they are of little use to the body and can impose serious health risks.

Fat

Although fatty foods, along with sugar, have been shown to damage good fat cells, not all fat that you eat is bad news. Tables have turned almost full circle when it comes to deciding what type of fat is considered beneficial in the diet and what's not. Even some forms of saturated animal fat, once considered a lethal weapon when it comes to cholesterol raising, have now been found to be not as damaging as was once thought.

Some fat is essential to include in the diet, while other types are best avoided if you want to stay healthy. So what's beneficial and what's best binned? There are basically three types of fat in the diet: saturated (mainly from animal sources), monounsaturated (such as the oils found in nuts, olive oil and avocado) and polyunsaturated (from plant foods and from oily fish). Nutritionists divide polyunsaturated fats into two groups of what they call essential fatty acids (or EFAs). It's crucial to have some in the diet because the body can't make them itself.

To help simplify the fat maze, here are some guidelines.

Include plenty of monounsaturated fats: hazelnuts, macadamia nuts, pecans, almonds, pistachios and cashews, olives, olive oil and avocado. Peanuts and peanut butter are also an excellent food source as are cashew and almond nut butters. Sesame seeds and sesame seed butter or paste – also known as tahini – are high in monounsaturated fatty acids. Sunflower seeds and sunflower seed butter, pumpkin and flaxseeds provide a smaller amount.

Aim to eat more omega-3 fatty acids: most people get too few of these in their diet. By far the best sources are oily fish like mackerel, herring and tuna. We can also get omega-3s in rapeseed, evening primrose and walnut oils, fresh seeds, especially hemp, pumpkin and sunflower, wholemeal bread and wholegrain breakfast cereals, leafy green vegetables and walnuts, but these provide omega-3 in a shorter chemical chain than oily fish which is more difficult for the body to convert into the beneficial compounds.

Don't eat too many omega-6 oils. Although we need them in our diet, most people get too many as they are widely present in processed and deep-fried foods. Sunflower and soybean and corn oil are sources as well as nuts and seeds.

Limit saturated fats. Saturated animal fats have had something of a bad rap, but scientists have now decided not all saturated fat is bad for us. When it comes in the form of dairy and lean red meat, some saturated fat might even be beneficial in the fight against heart disease. However, saturated fats are also found in biscuits, fatty cuts of meat and processed meats such as sausages and bacon – all sources that should be avoided.

Avoid trans fats. Of all the fats in modern food supplies, trans fats (or hydrogenated fats) are public enemy number one. Created when liquid oils are put through a rigorous chemical hydrogenation process to transform them into solids, they are considered more harmful to the heart and arteries than fat from any natural source. Their use is widespread in the food industry – they are present in margarines and spreads, biscuits and cakes, as well as ready meals and takeaways. They are cheap and tasty, but should be avoided. Not only do they appear to damage heart health, but they might impinge on the brain's synapses, affecting concentration.

Over-processing

As you've read, a calorie is not always a calorie, or at least not a calorie as you might understand it. The more processed a food – and we're not just talking manufacturing 'processes' to make ready meals here, but using highly refined ingredients such as white flour and rice and over-cooking homemade food – the more it can affect the energy value of a meal.

In short, soft, overcooked and highly processed foods require less effort to chew so you use up fewer calories digesting them. The more highly processed and overcooked a food, the more calories it provides. Likewise, foods with a high glycaemic index that are rapidly absorbed also entail less of a beneficial calorific slog by the body.

Conversely, the kind of lightly cooked, raw and fresh food along with low GI foods recommended in the Ice Diet generally require more chewing and are more difficult for the body to digest; you work harder to eat them. If you want to gain weight, make sure you eat highly processed and well-cooked meals as often as possible. To lose weight, do the opposite as outlined in the meal plans that follow.

Snacking

Snacking has long been considered a route to good health. Six or more mini-meals a day, we were told, were the best way to stabilize blood sugar, prevent cravings and, in turn, lose weight. But snacking habits have spiralled out of control. Our eating patterns, having altered beyond recognition in recent years, give people far greater access to food and reasons to stay up into the night, even if just to watch TV. And when people are awake, they tend to snack relentlessly. The result? It fuels the obesity problem.

As a result, science has changed its mind about multiple small snacks being the favourable option for shedding fat. Latest evidence points to less frequent meals being more beneficial for weight maintenance and fat loss. In one of the earlier trials, researchers from Purdue University in Indiana found overweight and obese men on low-calorie, high-protein diets felt more satisfied and less hungry when they ate three times a day compared to when they ate six times a day.[3] Lead researcher Dr Heather Leidy, now at the University of Missouri, said: 'These mini-meals everyone is talking about don't seem to be as beneficial as far as appetite control.'

Since then others have shown that, compared with constant snacking, two good meals a day is best for people with Type 2 diabetes – but could also benefit anyone trying to slim. A team of scientists from the Czech Republic asked volunteers to follow one of two diets, each containing 500 calories less than the recommended daily amount.[4] One group ate six small meals for twelve weeks, while the second group had a large meal at breakfast and lunchtime. Each group then switched regimens – both of which had the same macronutrient and calorie content – and continued for a further three months.

Measurements of liver-fat content, insulin sensitivity and the function of pancreatic beta cells – which produce insulin – were taken and the findings revealed that body weight fell in both diets – but there was a greater loss for those eating bigger meals. People eating twice a day lost around half a stone (3.7kg) during that period, compared with just over a quarter of a stone (2.3kg) for the snackers. Similar benefits were observed in substances that are critical to diabetics – there were better levels of chemicals such as the hormone glucagon and C-peptide, a protein involved in insulin synthesis, among people limited to two meals a day.

Foods to Limit on the Ice Diet

Ready meals
'White' foods: sugar, flour, pasta, rice, bread
Biscuits
Cakes
Processed meats: bacon, ham, pepperoni,
    Frankfurters, salami, sausages, canned meats
Refined breakfast cereals
Ready-made pasta sauces
Sugary soft drinks
Artificially sweetened desserts
Fruit juice/smoothies
Fizzy drinks
Margarines and spreads
Processed desserts
Flavoured yoghurts
Processed cheeses
Powdered milk
All foods containing trans fats
Bagged salads
Salted nuts and crisps
Canned meats
Commercial sauces and salad dressings

Putting It Right

Scheduled Eating

As we've seen in Chapter 2, a few trials have shown that mini-fasts involving careful mealtime scheduling are most likely to trigger good fat into action. There are other benefits to avoiding constant snacking on small meals. Scientists are increasingly convinced that stretching out the daily fasting period we naturally practise at night-time may override the adverse health effects of a high-fat diet and help to prevent obesity, diabetes and liver disease.

Our livers, intestines, muscles and other organs work to a metabolic cycle that is essential for good health. At certain times they operate at peak efficiency, but at other times they need rest. This 'sleep' period is critical for processes like cholesterol breakdown and glucose production to take place. Eating constantly throughout the day throws this metabolic cycle off-kilter.

We can prime our systems to turn on when we eat and back off when we don't, or vice versa. And scheduling mealtimes is one practical way to do that. It also has the added bonus of boosting good fat and helping us to eat less, both of which of course aid weight loss.

It's easier than you might think. Consider your current eating patterns and when you are most hungry. Really hungry, I mean, not peckish because you are bored. Then work out a meal-schedule ratio that will work for you. On the Ice Diet I recommend starting with a 12:12 – that's eating within a twelve-hour block of the day and avoiding food for the other twelve. For most people, this will mean eating your last meal no later than 8 p.m. so that you can then have breakfast in the morning.

Ideally you should eat two substantial meals a day, three if you are very active (or very hungry!), but certainly no more than that, with no snacking in between meals. I appreciate that switching to this approach from a diet that has seen you consume small meals regularly might be a psychological barrier but the generous portions in the Ice Diet will more than make up for the lack of a snack. As time goes on, I am sure that you will find you don't even think about them. I certainly found I snacked less and less as my body adapted to my meal schedule.

Once you feel comfortable with 12:12 (try it for at least two weeks), try to extend your 'fasting' period by an hour at a time with the ultimate aim of cutting the 'eating window' to between eight and ten hours. Much depends on when you prefer to eat your meals. Do not be swayed by commonly held beliefs that one meal is more important than another in terms of nutrition. For years we were told, for example, that breakfast would trigger our metabolism and aid our thinking powers. Breakfast-skippers were derided as flying in the face of nutritional science. But that's not the case. Several papers in the *American Journal of Clinical Nutrition* questioned whether there are any confirmed health benefits from eating first thing. In general, the consensus is that there's not; we can miss the morning meal without worrying about putting on weight. In one of the new studies, researchers at the University of

Alabama recruited nearly 300 volunteers who wanted to lose weight. They then randomly assigned each of them to follow one of three sets of dietary rules: stick to their current eating habits, cut out breakfast or eat an early-morning meal every day. After four months, the subjects returned to the Alabama labs to be weighed. Nobody had lost much weight and breakfast eaters fared no better on the scales than those who had skipped it.[5]

In another paper,[6] Dr James Betts, a researcher in nutrition and metabolism at the University of Bath, allocated a group of lean subjects to either a 'fasting' group or a 'breakfast' group for six weeks. Rules were simple: the fasting group were to consume no calories until 12 p.m. each day, with the breakfast group eating 350 calories within two hours of waking up and another 350 calories before 11 a.m. Measurements of their blood sugar, cholesterol levels and resting metabolic rates were taken and the volunteers were issued with an activity-tracking device. At the end of the trial, the breakfast eaters had experienced no improvements in snacking frequency or portion sizes or any change in their resting metabolism, contrary to popular opinion. There was one significant advantage from the morning meal – people who ate it moved around more, burning an extra 442 calories as a result. But don't forget they'd eaten more calories to start with, so it was more or less offset.

My point is that it doesn't matter which meal you skip. I'm a bruncher, not a breakfast eater, so actually prefer to postpone my first meal of the day until 10–11 a.m. I also find a 15:9 ratio suits my lifestyle best – taking my last meal at 7 or 8 p.m. and not eating until my 'brunch' the next day. Others I know prefer 14:10 (eat during ten hours of the day) or 16:8, which is initially tougher as you restrict your 'eating' hours to just eight. Experiment and don't worry if you get things wrong at first. The Ice Diet is intended to be a plan for life, not a short-term hardship.

Keep an Eye on the GI and the GL

The glycaemic index (GI) and glycaemic load (GL) of a food are systems of ranking foods based on how they affect blood sugar levels and insulin rise after they've been eaten. Originally developed to help people with diabetes control their blood glucose levels, the systems are now widely used by everyone from dieters to sports people as a means of determining which foods will provide the longest-lasting energy boost, thereby warding off hunger pangs and energy slumps. Generally, the lower a food's glycaemic index or glycaemic load, the less it affects blood sugar and insulin levels and the healthier an energy boost it is likely to provide.

High-GI foods and drinks – lemonade, white bread, cornflakes – will send blood sugar levels soaring. They are rapidly absorbed and cause a sharp rise in blood glucose levels, followed by a drop shortly afterwards. Preferable are low-GI foods, which are digested at a slower speed, making your blood glucose rise at a steady rate.

How much we eat of a food also has a huge influence on the effect it has on blood sugar. That's where the concept of the glycaemic load (GL) is based. The GL provides a value listed on the amount of a food you are likely to eat. Many foods that have high or medium GIs, such as kiwi fruit, pineapple and watermelon, can have low GLs because you are unlikely to gorge on them in huge amounts. But the worst offenders in the high-GI stakes – white rice, pasta, cornflakes and baked potato – are also likely to have high GLs, simply because we eat them to excess.

All GI figures are a value given to the food when it is prepared on its own. Add milk, sugar or honey to porridge (a low-GI food), for example, and it shifts the value somewhat. Neither the GI or GL tables are a hard-and-fast rule for what is healthy and what is not, but they are certainly a useful guide when it comes to food selection. On the Ice Diet, we limit the high-end value foods and focus on the lower GL/GI band – meaning longer-lasting energy bursts and fewer hunger pangs.

Table of GI and GL in Common Foods

FOOD	GI	SERVING SIZE	GL
SWEETS			
Honey	87	2 tbsp	17.9
Jelly Beans	78	25g	22
Table sugar (sucrose)	68	2 tsp	7
Strawberry jam	51	2 tbsp	10.1
BAKED GOODS & CEREALS			
Baguette	95	64g (1 slice)	29.5
Cornflakes	92	28g	21.1
Rice Krispies	82	33g	23
Bran Flakes	74	29g	13.3

Cheerios	74	30g	13.3
Bagel	72	89g	33
Wholemeal bread	70	28g (1 slice)	7.7
White bread	70	25g (1 slice)	8.4
Kellogg's Special K	69	31g	14.5
Croissant, butter	67	57g (1 med)	17.5
Bran muffin	60	113g (1 med)	30
Blueberry muffin	59	113g (1 med)	30
Porridge	58	117g	6.4
Wholewheat pitta	57	64g (1 pitta)	17
Popcorn	55	8g	2.8
Chocolate cake with icing	38	64g (1 slice)	12.5

DRINKS

Sports drink (powder)	78	16g scoop	11.7
Cranberry juice cocktail	68	253g	24.5
Fizzy cola	63	1 can	25.2
Orange juice	57	1 small glass	14.25
Pineapple juice	46	250g	14.7
Soy milk	44	245g	4
Apple juice	41	248g	11.9
Tomato juice	38	243g	3.4

PULSES AND LEGUMES

Baked Beans	48	253g	18.2
Chickpeas, Boiled	31	240g	13.3
Lentils	29	198g	7
Kidney Beans	27	256g	7
Soy Beans	20	172g	1.4
Peanuts	13	146g	1.6

(Continued)

Table of GI and GL in Common Foods (*Continued*)

FOOD	GI	SERVING SIZE	GL
VEGETABLES			
Potato	104	213g (1 med)	36.4
Parsnip	97	78g	11.6
Carrot, raw	92	15g (1 large)	1
Sweet Potato	54	133g	12.4
Peas, Frozen	48	72g	3.4
Tomato	38	123g (1 med)	1.5
Broccoli, cooked	0	78g	0
Cabbage, cooked	0	75g	0
Celery, raw	0	62g (1 stalk)	0
FRUIT			
Watermelon	72	152g	7.2
Pineapple, raw	66	155g	11.9
Cantaloupe melon	65	177g	7.8
Apricot, canned in light syrup	64	253g	24.3
Raisins	64	43g	20.5
Papaya	60	140g	6.6
Kiwi	58	76g (1 fruit)	5.2
Banana	51	118g (1 med)	12.2
Mango	51	165g	12.8
Orange	48	140g (1 fruit)	7.2
Grapes	43	92g	6.5
Strawberries	40	152g	3.6
Apples, w/ skin	39	138g (1 med)	6.2

Pears	33	166g (1 med)	6.9
Peach	28	98g (1 med)	2.2
Grapefruit	25	123g (½ fruit)	2.8
Plum	24	66g (1 fruit)	1.7
NUTS			
Cashews	26	50g	3.0
Peanuts	7	50g	0
MEAT/PROTEIN			
Most red meat	0–15	100g	0
Chicken	0–15	100g	0
Eggs	0–15	1 egg	0
Fish	0–15	100g	0
Lamb	0–15	100g	0
Pork	0–15	100g	0
Veal	0–15	100g	0
Venison	0–15	100g	0

Seasonal Foods

One of the best ways I've found to reconnect with natural cycles and monthly changes in temperature is to revert to eating in accordance with the seasons. This can be trickier than it sounds. So accustomed have we become to enjoying all-year-round availability of 'fresh' produce that it can take a bit of time and effort to reacquaint ourselves with what is actually seasonal and grown in the natural climates in which it thrives.

Less than one in ten people in one poll knew when

some of the best-known fruit and vegetables are in season.[7] At least 90 per cent of those surveyed could not name the correct months when produce such as broad beans, blackberries or asparagus are at their best. Even for one of the most popular seasonal fruits, strawberries, less than a quarter (23 per cent) knew that they were in season in June, July and August, suggesting the traditional rhythm of cooking and eating with the seasons is being lost.

Reverting to the practice of seasonal shopping and cooking does, I've found, bring benefits. It can add structure to your cooking and, of course, ensure the ingredients you use are as freshly harvested and as abundant with nutrients as they can be. Farm shops and, if you have the time, allotments are among the best ways to source these ingredients. Deliveries of organically grown vegetable boxes is another rapidly growing trend, although they tend to be more expensive than if you find the same fruit and vegetables grown locally.

The list below is by no means exhaustive, but gives an idea of how to eat according to the seasons:

WINTER (December, January, February)

Vegetables: beetroot, Brussels sprouts, cauliflower, celeriac, celery, chicory, horseradish, Jerusalem artichoke, kohlrabi, leeks, parsnips, cabbage, salsify, shallots, swede, turnip, kale, pak choi, pumpkin, radicchio, sweet potato
Fruit: apples, cranberries, blood oranges, grapefruit, dates,

quince, rhubarb, clementines, kiwi fruit, lemons, oranges, passion fruit, pears, pineapple, pomegranate, rhubarb, satsumas, tangerines, almonds, walnuts, Brazil nuts
Meat: turkey, venison, duck, autumn lamb, goose, pork
Fish: mussels, whiting, cod

SPRING (March, April, May)

Vegetables: Brussels sprouts, cabbage, cauliflower, celeriac, chicory, Jerusalem artichoke, leeks, new potatoes, pak choi, parsnips, peppers, purple sprouting broccoli, radicchio, sweet potato, spring greens, watercress, radishes
Fruit: bananas, nectarines, grapefruit, lemons, pomegranate, rhubarb, apricots
Meat: lamb, pork, venison
Fish: cod, halibut, crab, mackerel, salmon, tuna

SUMMER (June, July, August)

Vegetables: asparagus, aubergine, basil, beetroot, broccoli, cabbage, carrots, cavolo nero, celery, courgettes, courgette flower, fennel, garlic, globe artichoke, kohlrabi, lettuce, marrow, new potatoes, pak choi, peas, peppers, radicchio, radishes, samphire, spinach, Swiss chard, watercress
Fruit: apricots, bananas, blackberries, blackcurrants, cherries, figs, gooseberries, nectarines, peaches, pomegranate, raspberries, redcurrants, strawberries, tomatoes, watermelon
Meat: grouse, lamb, pork
Fish: crab, halibut, mackerel, salmon, tuna, whiting

AUTUMN (September, October, November)

Vegetables: aubergine, beetroot, broccoli, Brussels sprouts, cabbage, carrots, cavalo nero, celeriac, celery, courgettes, fennel bulb, garlic, globe artichoke, Jerusalem artichoke, kohlrabi, kale, lamb's lettuce, leeks, lettuce, pak choi, parsnips, peas, peppers, pumpkin, radicchio, runner beans, salsify, swede, sweet potato, Swiss chard, turnip, watercress
Fruit: apples, bananas, blackberries, clementines, cranberries, dates, figs, gooseberries, nectarines, pears, plums, pomegranate, raspberries, tomatoes
Meat: autumn lamb, duck, grouse, guinea fowl, pork, venison
Fish: crab, halibut, mackerel, mussels, whiting

Foods to Choose on the Ice Diet

Fresh, seasonal fruits – especially apples, cranberries, bilberries
Prunes
Herbs – especially basil, peppermint, rosemary, lavender, oregano, thyme
Peppers – red, yellow and chilli peppers
Porridge oats
Lean meat
Fish and seafood – especially oily fish like mackerel, herring, tuna, etc.
Avocados
Nuts and seeds
Olive, walnut and flaxseed oils
Plain yoghurt

Fresh, seasonal vegetables
Eggs
Grains – quinoa, barley, brown rice, wild rice
Legumes – chickpeas, lentils, beans

Drinks

Ice-cold water
Unsweetened icy drinks
Milk
Green tea
Black tea

What to Have in Moderation

Alcohol
Coffee – black or with added milk
Diet drinks
Dried fruits
Wholegrain pasta
Bread
Cereals

Practical Tips – How to Prepare Your Food

Over-cooked and over-processed food provides more calories than lightly cooked food because it is softer and
easier for the body to digest. You also lose out on valuable
vitamins and minerals. There's no need to avoid cooking
altogether (although some raw foods recipes are fantastic), just to use healthier preparation techniques.

Steaming

Veggies and fish are great for steaming – it allows them to cook quickly and retain natural goodness. Too much heat can break down 15–20 per cent of nutrients in some foods, particularly vitamin C and potassium, so fast techniques are preferable

Boiling and Poaching

Make sure the water you use is boiling when you add the food you are cooking and these approaches can be quick. A downside is that water-soluble vitamins (A, C and E) can be leeched. Poaching (cooking in a small amount of fluid) is a very gentle way to prepare fruit, eggs and fish.

Stir-frying

A great way to cook bite-sized pieces of vegetables and meat. You need very little oil and, on a high heat, a dish can be prepared in minutes.

Microwaving

This approach has come into its own after previously being considered a way to nuke your food. Studies have shown that microwaving vegetables is one of the best ways to preserve their nutrient content. One paper[8] found that microwaved vegetables retained 90 per cent of their vitamin C compared to 22–34 per cent of vitamins and minerals preserved when they were boiled or steamed.

Un-cooking

Raw fruits and vegetables are at no risk of nutrients being lost or of calories being added by decreasing the energy required to chew. Having said that, not all foods are better raw: the amount of the beneficial antioxidant substance lycopene is amplified when tomatoes are cooked. Likewise, the health-boosting carotenoid compounds in carrots, peppers and sweet potatoes increases after cooking.

Limit juicing and pulping

Smoothies have become hugely popular in recent years, but when it comes to calories they are not such a healthy idea. Juice disciples say that the tough, fibrous cell walls on fruits and vegetables can hamper the digestion of nutrients by the body. Breaking those cell walls down can prevent that, they claim. But by the time we eat or drink liquefied fruit and vegetables, they are almost mechanically pre-chewed, which spares your body the energy it would have used to get it to that stage.

How to Keep Your Cool

Any new health programme requires a degree of change and the Ice Diet is no different in that respect. And while it's designed to pose minimal challenges, there will inevitably be times when you struggle more than others to make the healthy switches. So how do you keep your cool and keep it up?

Make gradual changes: When it comes to your meal-scheduling, don't plunge into the 16:8 approach thinking it will have the greatest weight-loss effect. If you are not used to longish periods without food, then you'll be more likely to snack. As recommended, start with the 12:12 ratio and gradually extend the mini-fasting period. Make it work for you.

Expect hunger: Part of the problem with modern diets and the trend for constant snacking is that we no longer recognize real hunger. We think we are hungry when we are thirsty. Or bored. As you adapt to your new pattern, you will experience hunger pangs, but learn to accept them as a good thing, only succumbing when they are overwhelming. You might get more hungry when you initially add the cooling strategies discussed in the next chapter, so be prepared for this too.

Enjoy food and look forward to it: We are not talking deprivation on the Ice Diet. Healthy, tasty food is an important part of the plan. There's no counting calories or obsessing over different food groups – the idea is to enjoy what you are consuming in your scheduled window of eating.

Adapt it: The rules of the Ice Diet are not set in stone. It's recommended that you eat two or three meals a day. If you are highly active, you may veer towards three rather than two a day and need a boost after your workout. This approach is designed to be flexible and to morph with your lifestyle.

Don't lose heart: You are not a failure if you eat more than you intended on a particular day. Likewise, you will not relinquish the benefits gained from previous days of eating well from a twenty-four-hour slip. Start afresh the next morning.

Ice Diet Rules

- Eat preferably two but a maximum of three meals a day. More active people should aim for three.
- Eat only within your scheduled meal 'window'.
- Avoid snacking – only resort to a healthy and small snack if you really feel hungry, not because you are bored.
- Avoid refined and 'white' foods; aim for low GI rather than high GI.
- Cut down your sugar intake and the sugary foods you consume.
- Flavour food with chilli and spices when you can – not only do they taste more appetizing,

but they can stimulate appetite and the activity of 'good fat'.

- Cook lightly – steam, sauté, stir-fry, fast boil.
- Don't over-process your diet – that means less processed and ready-made foods as well as less juicing and pulping, mashing and grinding. Eat whole fruits and vegetables as opposed to juices and smoothies.
- Drink cold water flavoured with lemon and lime; no fizzy or sweetened drinks.
- Embrace the seasons – eat the foods that are in season.

5 Preparing to Acclimatize

There are, as we've seen, some convincing reasons to cool your lifestyle. Many will take effect immediately. You may sleep better, feel more alert and energetic during the day. Less central heating will have a positive effect on your skin, which will feel less dry and papery. Other effects become evident over time.

You will, of course, be boosting the rate at which your body burns calories by activating good fat. And that, inevitably, will lead to weight loss provided you also stick to the kind of healthy eating plan and exercise that is outlined in the next few chapters. And there are plentiful health benefits to boot.

With the compelling evidence for cooler living, it's now time to put things into practice. Having shown why it works, in this chapter I'll reveal in more detail how to go about reducing everyday temperatures without it impacting on your enjoyment of life, including tips from my own experiences of living with less heat. It's not intended to be a sharp shock approach. Make the changes gradually and I promise you won't feel too cold, just all the better for it.

Of course, none of it will work unless you have the backing of the rest of the household. It's no good announcing that you have read *The Ice Diet* and there will be no heating on until December. There must be a gradual period of acclimatization. It took a while to train my partner into having what I termed 'healthy air flow' in our bedroom in deepest mid-winter, but he eventually adjusted.

I found it amusing to read that how hot a home should be is the top cause of family squabbles. One in four adults apparently has an argument about the central heating, with four in ten women admitting they have secretly cranked it up without telling their partner.[1] Of those who admitted having heated arguments, nearly three-quarters say they argued over the temperature of the house and nearly one-quarter over what date the heating should go on in winter.

Obviously I do not want this book to be the source of family discord or relationship quibbles, so my advice is to present your evidence about the benefits of keeping it low, resist the early 'switch-on' and stand your ground when the rest of the family say they would prefer to be walking around indoors in their T-shirts from autumn through to spring.

At Home

Since learning about the benefits of cooler living on good fat and calorie burning, I have to say I've developed something of a central-heating fixation at home. I don't go as far as seeing my own breath indoors, but like to keep it low for as long as I can. My barometer for a healthy temperature is that our home should always be cool enough to warrant a jumper in winter.

It's an obsession that can rear itself in unusual ways when I visit someone else's greenhouse-hot home. The more artificially heated a house is, the more I find myself questioning how healthy its inhabitants are. Doctors swear that as soon as central heating goes on, so their waiting rooms become crammed with patients with runny noses, streaming eyes and sore throats. And I vividly remember how healthy we were as children living in what was, in retrospect, a chilly home with draughts whistling through the ill-fitting windows.

I am certainly not advocating no heating at all. We live in the modern world. We are not Stone-Agers and there's no doubt that technological advancements in heating have helped to save lives, particularly among the elderly. It's just that we have now got too hot and need to adjust to using it with more thought and consideration. There are other ways to conserve heat without making your home stiflingly hot.

Drawing curtains or pulling blinds at dusk in the winter months will reduce draughts without having to turn up the heating dial and, if you do have the central heating on, make sure you keep it low or at least don't have the room too warm. Not covering radiators with clothing or blocking them with furniture further increases their efficiency.

I've found that hourly changes helped us to get used to going lower. Keeping moderately warm for an hour, then turning the thermostat down a few notches for ten minutes or so is far more bearable in the early stages than going straight for the minimal figures on the dial. It's astonishing how easily the body adjusts to cooling when it is taken in barely perceptible stages. Remember, there are financial as well as health benefits: turning down heating by just 1 °C (1.8 °F) could save up to 10 per cent on your fuel bills, not to mention the boost you will get to good fat and calorie burning.

In the Bathroom

Certainly, there is no need to inflict torture upon yourself every morning by switching the dial to blue. In fact, I would advise against very cold showers – too uncomfortable, too shocking to the system – and argue in favour of slightly cooler. Even for someone like me who was an avid fan of steaming baths and showers that would almost scald as I got in them, causing my legs to redden, gradually lowering the water temperature was tolerable.

By adjusting and turning down the heat over several weeks, I found myself washing in water that was altogether cooler. Even more surprisingly, I didn't find it a hardship. Some people swear by going the whole way. One 'good fat' researcher I spoke to told me he has been taking cold showers for six years and believes they are helpful in prompting calorie burning. It might be worth the bravery, but rather him than me.

There is no need to become completely masochistic about cold showering. I now prefer a cool 1–2-minute blast at the end of a warm shower. Or a 'contrast' shower in which you finish with fast 10-second bursts of warm, then cold. This approach was recommended to me by Ray Cronise, who repeats the process ten times. I prefer a shorter shower session of 5×10-second bursts. Like exercise, it takes time to train yourself to adjust to this kind of sharp shock (and it's not recommended for anyone with heart problems or on medication). When you do, it can make a difference. Of course, it is up to you when you choose to shower – there is no wrong or right time to do it. Ray says he often showers this way just before going to sleep at night.

There are plenty who believe that icy cold is the way to go. Celebrity trainer Jon Denoris recommends his clients fill a basin with ice-cold water and put their feet in it for up to 15 minutes first thing in the morning. 'It's definitely one for the brave and hardy,' he warns. He also recommends the contrast or 'rotation' shower as a less daunting option. 'Take a shower for 5 minutes, alternating 20 seconds cold, 10 seconds room temperature,' Denoris advises.[2]

Ultimately, how you shower must come down to preference. An icy shower might offer minimal gains in terms of weight loss (although, as yet, there is no confirmed proof), but I prefer the more comfortable, enjoyable route to cooling.

In the Office

An advantage for me of being a home-worker is that I can control the temperature of my working environment, and step outside whenever I feel the need for some fresh air.

But what of those who are office-based and have to endure the sometimes stifling conditions to which many people are exposed at their place of work? Millions of office workers don't know when the sun is shining and have no idea how warm or cold it is outside much of the time.

How can you tell if your workplace is too hot? In the UK, the Health and Safety Executive issues guidelines which place a legal obligation on employers to provide a 'reasonable' temperature. That is deemed to be a minimum temperature of 16 °C, or 13 °C if much of the work indoors involves severe physical effort. They are not absolute legal requirements; it's down to an employer to determine what's reasonably comfortable for the staff.

But you can push for change. If more than 10–15 per cent of employees complain that an office is too hot (or indeed too cold) much of the time, then the HSE suggests it might be necessary to carry out a 'thermal comfort' risk assessment. Of course, there is no pleasing everybody. When office managers turn up the indoor temperature because it is cold outside, they'll get a complaint from Julie in Marketing who says she is sweltering. If they turn it down, it'll be Mark in Human Resources complaining his fingers and toes are numb.

If practicable, cooler work spaces are obviously going to be more beneficial when it comes to increasing your calorie burn and the activity of good brown fat. At home, it goes without saying that it is best to work in a cool room, putting on an extra pair of socks instead of the heating.

Clothing

It struck me quite how used we have become to wearing more clothes than we really need when I was watching my nine-year-old son play football last year. It was a crisp autumnal morning, warm enough to melt the frost that had been on the ground first thing and with clear blue skies overhead. There was no breeze and the ground had lost its icy hardness well before we arrived for the 10 a.m. kick-off. It was a perfect day to be outside – chilly, but certainly not catch-your-breath cold.

Yet when the teams took to the pitches, most children were wearing so many clothes that I doubt they were aware of the bite in the air. Almost without exception, they were dressed in base layers and thermal leggings beneath the football kit. Some wore gloves and hats. One had on a thick fleece and the goalkeeper had to squeeze his bib over a bulky quilted anorak.

What, I wondered, would they be wearing when there was a proper cold snap, when a freezing wind and soft snowflakes rendered the chill factor less bearable? Of course, children are less able to tolerate extremes in temperatures than adults, but this was far from a drop in temperature that might put them at risk. And if they were cocooned against the elements on a day when they didn't need extra layers, how would they acclimatize when it really got cold?

When it comes to sport and leisure activities, much of the emphasis on the need to dress excessively warmly has come, unsurprisingly perhaps, from clothing manufacturers. In the two decades I have worked as a health and fitness journalist, a job that involves testing and reviewing many of these advances in design, the development of technological fabrics designed to trap heat and repel water, to wick away sweat and protect us from the elements, ensuring we never get really cold, has exploded beyond all expectation.

Top footballers have taken to wearing snoods, leggings and gloves. Arm warmers are another new invention regularly worn by the sporting elite, as are knee-length 'compression' socks, supposed to prevent muscle fatigue as well as keep you warm. It wasn't until I watched my son and his friends play on that bright autumn morning that I realized I am as guilty as the next person of layering up beyond my needs. I'm a lifelong runner. I took up the sport at eleven and am still plodding along more than three decades on. Before thermal fabrics were invented and before heat panels were added to tops and leggings, I would run in shorts all year round without a second thought because nothing else was available.

In the intervening years I had layered up like everyone else. I found myself heading out for a run on a winter morning dressed as if for an Arctic expedition. I had a merino wool thermal base layer underneath a long-sleeved bamboo-based running top, full-length running leggings with a waterproof outer layer, thermal sweat-wicking gloves, a fleece headband, a 'breathable' and waterproof jacket, insulated running socks and waterproof trainers. I was impenetrable. But did I need it all? Of course not.

Within minutes of setting out I was always too warm and was stripping off layers much faster than I had put them on. Of course, sometimes more clothing is necessary. In a cold snap I like the fact that I can wear long or three-quarter-length leggings. But my point is that we should layer up within reason. We have been convinced, largely through clever marketing, that we need to dress for extreme weather conditions as soon as summer is over. Not just when we are being active, but in our everyday lives.

We pile on the gilets and duck-down jackets, the ski gloves and hats at the first sign of a temperature drop, only to discover we are overheating ourselves. Far better to carry additional layers if you suspect you might need them than to put on too much and over-insulate. Within reason, your body is adept at maintaining its core temperature. And it has a well-tuned cold indicator that will signal when you really do need to wrap up – shivering.

Think carefully about what you put on and whether you really need to wear it. I've lost count of the times I've been out in sheepskin-lined boots only to find that my feet were sweltering as I walked around overheated shops. Now I am much more of a minimalist dresser. I dress for how I'll feel 10 minutes after leaving the house, not for the initial cold blast that hits you as you first walk out the door. It's been a revelation and it really pays off in terms of calorie burning.

Protect Your Extremities

Given my thoughts about the trend for wearing too many layers, you might think I am of the opinion that we should forsake all warming accessories. Well, no. What I've discovered is that we need to cover up strategically, to expose parts of the body that aren't prone to frostbite, but to protect those that are more vulnerable to the effects of really cold temperatures.

You may recall how Stamford University researchers discovered that our body's core temperature can be controlled by manipulating the exposure of our hands, face and feet to heat. In these areas, we have in-built radiators packed with a network of veins that can carry varying amounts of blood flow. Our bodies shut down blood flow to these extremities when they detect cold and you effectively enter the early stages of survival mode.

It is these areas that are more prone to frostbite and which, in extreme conditions, should be the first we protect by donning earmuffs or hat, gloves and warm socks. The trunk is better equipped to cope with temperature drops and reacts to the cold by producing heat, activating good fat and burning up calories.

The Ice Rules

Reasons for avoiding unnecessarily high temperatures in your daily life are plentiful. Here are the Ice Rules for cooler living.

Turn Down the Thermostat

Resist turning on the heating in autumn until it's absolutely necessary. And when you do, keep it lower than usual. About 19 °C is as high as your heating needs to go. Get used to it by adjusting in increments. Turn down the heating by a notch (1 °C) – just that amount could also save 10 per cent on your fuel bills.

Open a Window

Airtight double glazing creates a warm, stifling environment that is of absolutely no use to our bodies when it comes to fat burning. Even if you do it once an hour and for only 5–10 minutes in the winter, let the cooler air in.

Sleep in a Cooler Room

Reduce the tog of your duvet if needed and open a window. A bedroom cooled to a perfectly reasonable 19 °C has been found to stimulate brown fat and trigger the body to burn more calories into daylight hours.

Take a Cooler Shower

This sounds hardcore, but in reality a cold blast at the end of the shower will suffice. Try a 5-minute warm (not scorching) shower followed by 2 or 3 minutes of cool water to get used to the lower temperature. Don't, however, do it to the point of discomfort. As you get used to the lower temperature, try a contrast shower in which you shower for several minutes in warm (not hot) water and towards the end alternate between 10 seconds of warm, 10 seconds of cold. Repeat as often as you like, up to ten times.

Switch Temperatures

Our good fat responds best to changes in indoor temperature without ever letting rooms get too hot. We can easily tolerate changes of 2 °C per hour, so alternate the temperature in your room from around 16 °C to 19 °C every 60 minutes.

Get Outside

There is no better place to get good brown fat doing what it is good at than the great outdoors. Make a concerted effort to spend at least the equivalent of 5–10 minutes for every one of your waking hours outdoors. For most people that is around 1–2 hours a day.

Change your Workout Environment

Easy if you work from home, more tricky if you work in a large office. But canvas your colleagues and see if you can negotiate a less stuffy office by lowering the thermostat a notch or two for at least some of the day.

Watch What You Wear

Protect your extremities in very cold weather, but don't layer up beyond your needs. Prioritize earmuffs or a hat, gloves and socks rather than woolly jumpers and fleecy layers. When exercising, remember that you will get warmer than you were when you first set out within a relatively short time. Wear what is a sensible amount of clothing, but avoid unnecessary layers.

Cool Blasts

One of my favourite means of cold exposure is through short, sharp blasts of cold air. You can achieve this simply by stepping outside on a frosty day or by opening a window. Some people prefer the icy blast of a short shower, hand or footbath. All help you to acclimatize to cooler living.

Live According to the Seasons

A simple rule of thumb I like to stick to is never to walk around the house in a T-shirt when the heating is on. If you can do this, it is too hot. Way too warm, in fact. Get back in touch with the fact that it is autumn or winter, it is meant to be colder and you are supposed to throw on a jumper or cardigan to keep warm. Humans were not designed to be oven-ready.

6 Getting Ready

You are about to embark on more than a healthy eating plan. The Ice Diet, backed by dozens of scientific trials, prescribes lifestyle changes for the better. Given that it is an approach to stick to for life, I have made it easy to adopt. There's no complicated elimination of entire food groups, no totting up of calories and no starvation.

Schedule your eating hours, then follow the nutritional guidelines outlined in Chapter 8 and use the delicious and nutrient-packed meal plans and recipes that follow and you will find your weight and vitality quickly transformed.

Healthy eating is the essential bedrock of the Ice Diet, but as you have seen, it is only part of the story. Metabolism-boosting enhancements come in the form of the ice strategies that have been shown to increase calorie burning, activate good body fat and enable you to reap other benefits such as more energy, lower risk of obesity and all-round excellent good health.

None of this need happen overnight. Years of eating and living habits take time to change and my advice is not to rush things. Acclimatize gradually to your new way of living. First things first: get your diet in order so that snacking is minimal or obsolete and your body adapts to consuming satiating and varied foods.

Then, and only then, complete the transition by gradually

cooling your daily life, spending more time outdoors and living as nature intended. It should never be torturous and you should never think of yourself as a failure if you occasionally fall off the Ice Diet wagon. All of us have moments of weakness. In the grand scheme of things, an occasional dietary slip-up is small fry compared with a lifetime of eating unhealthily.

When to Start

There is no time like the present. Of course, there are always reasons *not* to make the switch to a healthier way of living. You might think you are too busy, too tired or too stressed to take the plunge, but really, what's stopping you? Part of the joy of the Ice Diet is that you can look forward to feeling brimful of vitality through eating wholesome food. You will not feel hungry. And, since the cooling strategies are adopted slowly, it will take barely any extra effort to burn additional calories without realizing it.

As with any diet, there are precautions of which you need to be aware. Always have a health check with your doctor before trying any new eating or lifestyle programme. If you have any underlying medical condition or have an eating disorder, then you should not follow any diet other than that prescribed by your own medical team.

And while a cooler lifestyle is definitely an advantage for children, they should never be subjected to an eating plan that restricts food in any way. Children are growing and, contrary to trials on adults, studies have shown that their bodies and brains thrive on regular, top-notch nutrition, including breakfast.

For the rest of you, though, now is as good a time as any to get started. Here's to a cooler new you.

Set Your Meal Schedule

Right, we are now down to the business end of the preparation. Remember that the Ice Diet is based on 'meal scheduling', an approach that has been shown in clinical trials to have plentiful health benefits, not least the activation of good fat, the boosting of your metabolism and weight loss.

Take a long hard look at your current eating habits. Over five days, keep a food journal and jot down not *what* you eat, but *when* you consume food and, importantly, *why* you do it. Be brutally honest with yourself. If that blueberry muffin was a social event rather than a means to stopping your stomach from eating itself in response to hunger, then say so. If you wake ravenously hungry and can't face the day without filling your stomach, then write it down.

From your notes you will be able to establish a rough idea of when your body most needs food. For me it is mid-morning and early evening, although I do shift my evening meal back a couple of hours to around 8 p.m. so that I can eat with my partner. It might be that you prefer an early breakfast and an earlier evening meal. Another rule:

don't sacrifice relationships and home happiness for the sake of your diet.

Once you have an idea of when you like to have your meals, the next step is to establish your own meal schedule, the window during which you should try to eat each day. Generally, my recommendation is to start with a 12:12 ratio – that's three meals consumed within 12 hours. If you can reduce that to two daily meals, all the better.

After a few weeks, you will probably discover that any hunger pangs (which happen largely through boredom) have disappeared. That might be the time to reassess your meal scheduling. Chop no more than an hour off your window and allow your body plenty of time to adapt. Ultimately, you are looking to extend the 'mini-fasting' period to 14–16 hours and narrow your eating window accordingly.

Again, I must stress that this is not intended to be a life sentence. If it's too difficult, revert to the 12:12 option and try to obliterate snacking. Follow the meal plans and your body (and mind) will benefit anyway. The worst thing you can do is beat yourself up about eating – it will simply set off a nasty spiral of negative thoughts. Life is just too short for all of that.

Set Your Cooling Strategies

When it comes to the practicalities of implementing cooling strategies, there is only one way to do it: gradually. My advice is to adapt no more than one cooling approach a week and to allow your body to get accustomed to it before moving on to add the next. Do it properly and you will barely notice it, let alone experience any discomfort.

I started in winter when it was easy to turn the central heating down a notch. It's amazing how quickly your body acclimatizes to these small adjustments in temperature. Over the course of several weeks, I lowered the temperature in our house from a sweltering 23 °C to 19 °C without anyone complaining they felt chilly.

For cold blasts, you have several options: lower the temperature on the central heating by a few degrees (or turn it off) for 10–20 minutes in the winter, open a window for some icy airflow or workout outside (a walk is as good as anything) instead of at the stifling gym. You can also get an ice blast with contrast showers (a few minutes of cooler water at the end or 10 seconds warm, 10 seconds cold at the end of a warm shower).

At night, gradually introduce cooling strategies. Open a window, use a lighter duvet or just a sheet if it is very warm. I now rarely have any heating in the bedroom and sleep much more comfortably as a result. And then there's clothing. On colder days, do not over-layer. By all means carry extra fleeces and jumpers with you, but don't put them on just because you fear getting cold.

It is, in fact, quite liberating to realize that your body adjusts to temperatures and that you do not suffer in the way you think. Like hunger, our over-warming is as much a learned behaviour and a force of habit as anything else. We evolved without needing to be permanently toasty and we can unlearn our reliance on it more easily and pain-lessly than you imagine.

Tracking Your Progress

It's by no means essential to measure and track your pro-gress, but knowing that things are heading in the right direction can be hugely motivational. There's nothing like feeling you have stalled on the weight- or fat-loss front only to step on the scales and find that the reading is more positive than you thought.

Self-monitoring is hugely popular and expensive devices are available to measure everything from the number of seconds you spend moving and the level of effort entailed to hours spent sleeping and calories burned. If you buy into this daterati trend, fine. If not, there are simpler (and far cheaper) means of keeping check on how your body is responding to the Ice Diet.

None are compulsory, but I find that keeping a note of measurements in my diary can be inspirational.

BMI: I've included this measure because it is by far the most widely used. However, I am not a fan. It is a rudimentary formula that has somehow exceeded all expectations when it comes to its own popularity. Devised by the Belgian statistician Adolphe Quetelet, it has been used to define weight for over a century. It's been adopted by hospitals and doctors' surgeries, insurance companies, university researchers, drugs companies and slimming clubs; and many professions require prospective employees to have a BMI that does not exceed healthy recommendations. Part of its appeal is that it's so simple to work out: weight in kilograms is divided by height in metres squared. Someone with a BMI of less than 18.5 is considered underweight, between 18.5 and 24.9 is 'normal', 25 to 29.9 is 'overweight' and 30 or greater is clinically obese.

It's simple, but the downfall of BMI is that it does not take into account either gender or body composition – whether or not excess weight is fat or muscle – which is why athletes and the super-fit often find themselves in a less desirable category of the BMI rating system. I know people who are highly athletic, with barely an ounce of visible fat on their Amazonian bodies, yet they are officially plump when they calculate their BMI. From Olympians to the likes of Brad Pitt, who was considered 'overweight' during his *Fight Club* prime, the BMI calculation can deliver a damning blow.

It can also produce skewed results in studies. Studies that have looked at the accuracy and usefulness of the BMI have found that while severely obese patients had a higher risk of death, overweight people had fewer heart problems than those with a normal BMI because the inaccuracies meant that many of the 'overweight' were in fact fit and muscular. The long and short of it is that the BMI should be used with caution. If you are Joe Average, you can use the Body Mass Index equation as a vague approximation of fatness, but nothing more. If you are supremely fit or even on the periphery of gym body status, then you are best to forget it.

Tape measure: Just because outdated measurements

of relative fatness like the BMI are no longer considered helpful in assessing a healthy body shape, it doesn't mean you should throw away the tape measure. An emerging new favourite is the 'waist: half height' ratio. The idea is to measure your waist circumference and make sure that figure is always equal to or less than half your height. For a 6ft man, this would mean having a waistline smaller than 36in, while a 5ft 4in woman should have a waist size no larger than 32in. Keeping your waist circumference to less than half your height can help prevent the onset of conditions like stroke, heart disease and diabetes and add years to life. It's been shown to be a far better predictor of life expectancy than BMI by researchers at Oxford Brookes University.[1]

Pedometer: A useful buy when you come to incorporate the exercise outlined in Chapter 8. A basic pedometer costs as little as five pounds, but it can match an expensive fitness tracker when it comes to motivating people to move more. A study at Indiana University asked men and women between the ages of 40 and 66 to stick to a twelve-week programme in which they wore a cheap pedometer every day. They were encouraged to be active at times they would normally spend sitting (at a desk, in front of the TV) and to download the data once a week. Results were impressive: they spent a lot less time sitting and more time being active, dropping an average of 2.5 pounds in weight.

Scales: Weighing yourself daily remains one of the most effective motivators to weight loss. Jessica LaRosse, Assistant Professor of Behavioural Health at Virginia

Commonwealth University School of Medicine, conducted a study[2] including 178 overweight volunteers who were randomly assigned one of two calorie-reduced diets. Both groups were also asked to do at least 200 minutes a week of activity. During the eighteen-month study some people were more diligent than others at the daily scale-hopping. Ultimately, though, those who weighed themselves every day lost more weight. 'Stepping on the scales every day provides immediate and concrete information about how eating and activity impact your weight,' LaRosse said. 'It cues you to make changes to stay on track with your goals.'

Body Fat: If anything, this is the most accurate measure of fatness. There are several approaches to body-fat testing and if you have ever joined a gym, you will be familiar with the skin calliper tests that pinch your fat folds. It's uncomfortable and notoriously difficult to perform if someone is very overweight, but they can give an accurate reading if done properly. Fat tests can be skewed by things such as thicker skin on men's backs and it will take a few tests to gain an accurate average. For home use, you can buy body-fat scales that provide an estimate of your body-fat percentage and work by sending a very small current through the body when you stand on the scales, but their accuracy varies. They are less accurate than the calliper test, but more convenient. Once you have your body-fat percentage, you can use the figure to determine whether you need to shift any weight. These figures are useful guidelines.[3]

	WOMEN	MEN
Essential fat	10–12%	2–4%
Athletes	14–20%	6–13%
Fitness	21–24%	14–17%
Acceptable	25–31%	18–25%
Obese	32% plus	26% plus

What NOT to Expect on the Ice Diet

As you've seen, the Ice Diet requires some overhauling not only of the food you eat, but the way you live. Any new approach to food might be regarded with some trepidation. Will it make you hungry? Tired and irritable? How challenging will it be and will the result be worthwhile? One or all of these factors are usually the reason why people have ditched diets in the past. For it to work, a healthy eating programme must fuse seamlessly with your lifestyle otherwise the 'stickability' will be woefully short. So, what not to expect on the Ice Diet? Here goes:

Overwhelming hunger: If you are the kind of person who currently sticks to the six or more small meals a day rule, then adjusting to the scheduled eating plans advocated here could take a little longer than for someone who is more accustomed to, say, three meals a day. However, most people find it much easier than they think to cut down, particularly when they are consuming the delicious and nutrient-dense food recommended in the plans. Also, your body loves consistency, which is why a carefully planned meal schedule in which you are eating at around the same times every day can go a long way in regulating appetite. When your meals are all over the place, it's much easier to confuse true hunger with boredom or other emotions. And then comes the urge to snack. That cycle can be broken by eating within your 'window'.

One point worth mentioning here is that getting too cold too quickly and for too long will spur a degree of calorie burning that can trigger hunger. This is another reason to adopt cooling strategies slowly.

Feeling uncomfortably cold: It's been stressed throughout the book that this is not the aim of the Ice Diet. If it is to be effective, adaptation to cold must be progressive, starting with the smallest increments of cold exposure and temperature change. You will be surprised how quickly you adapt, though. How a walk on a crisp autumn day that would once have seen you bundled up like the Michelin Man, now requires you to layer up minimally. And how refreshing and invigorating you find it to expose your body to blasts of cold air or water. It's because you are reconnecting with Nature's blueprint and living as was intended.

It will be stressful: One of the downfalls of most diets is that, the minute you start, you become obsessed with calories, food groups and the weighing scales. A reason they fail is because you are forced to narrow your outlook on life: suddenly everything you do revolves around what and when you eat. Not so on the Ice Diet. It is less rigid, more flexible. Yes, you will lose weight, but with emphasis also on cooling strategies and being active, the focus is not solely on avoiding food. And by adopting these other means of improving your health, studies show that the whole dieting experience is less stressful. Researchers at Laval University in Québec, Canada, showed that by reducing the focus on food restriction and weight loss and indicating other positive things participants could do to improve their health, they were able to help volunteers avoid the stress related to weight loss. In their trial, those who were told to adopt healthy living techniques rather than just 'to diet' showed significantly less 'food disinhibition' or losing control around food during stress or other situations that trigger overeating.[4]

Weight gain: Almost certainly you will experience the opposite, finding that your belt needs tightening after just a few weeks. A pleasant side effect for me is that, as I live more healthily according to Ice Diet rules, my body and taste buds have developed an innate preference for healthy foods. I no longer crave sugary carbs and my reliance on extra-strong espressos for a boost has also diminished. I am pretty sure you will find the same thing happens to you. There is growing evidence that the meal-schedule windows are a fantastic way to shed weight.

You want to give up: This is the least likely scenario. Given that you will not feel hungry or tired on this plan, that your health will improve along with your weight and appearance, the motivation to continue is, in many ways, ready made. It's worth stressing again how important it is to get your diet in order before adding cooling. Studies show that people who set too many goals at the same time, such as trying to quit smoking while dieting, are more likely to fail at both than people who tackle them at a more sensible pace.

A lot comes down to willpower and self-control. A psychologist friend of mine says that willpower is like a muscle and that you can train it to respond positively at times when you might be vulnerable – when the dough-nuts appear at work, for example. One tip she gave me to speed up our self-control recovery, or give it a boost when reserves are low, is simply to think about people you know who have lots of self-control. It's astounding the differ-ence it can make to call to mind a friend who always says 'no' when the cakes come round, and who looks all the better for it. A pick-me-up can also help. Anything that makes you feel good – in my case, a run, a coffee with friends, a shopping trip – can help to restore your self-control strength when you're looking for a quick posi-tivity fix.

7 The 6-Week Ice Diet Plan

The Food

Remember that the key is to set your meal schedule and eat your meals within that window. Start with a 12:12 window: that's three meals a day during twelve hours. As your eating window narrows, reduce the daily meals to two unless you are very active. Choose any two meals: brunch and dinner, breakfast and lunch, lunch and dinner and so on. The following schedule is a useful guideline, but don't reduce either your meal window or the number of meals too hastily. It will result in miserable hunger pangs and a downturn in mood – not what you are after.

Weeks 1 and 2

Schedule your meals within a 12:12 ratio (that's a twelve-hour eating window). Start with three meals a day.

Weeks 3 and 4

Schedule your meals within a 13:11 ratio (that's an eleven-hour eating window). Experiment on two days with just two meals. Revert to three if it proves too challenging for now.

Weeks 5 and 6

Schedule your meals within a 14:10 or 15:9 ratio (that's a ten- or nine-hour eating window). Make the shift towards two meals on three days if you feel comfortable with that. If not, stay at three until (and only when) you find it manageable.

The Cooling

You will notice that cooling strategies are added daily throughout the six weeks. In reality, there is no set structure and you can add more cooling as you feel fit. Remember, the golden rule is that all cooling strategies should be tolerable – don't dive into anything too cold, too soon. Don't adopt another cooling strategy until you have successfully adapted to the current one. It can take time even to adjust to opening a window an hour before you go to bed on a cool winter evening. There is no rush to 'complete' the Ice Diet and it is better to adopt long-term cooler living than to be put off by too much shivering in the early days.

The Activity

Regular activity is crucial for overall health and I've included a daily activity recommendation, aimed at those who are moderately active, to complement the Ice Diet programme. It is by no means obligatory and if you have not exercised in a while, or spend much of your time sitting down at a desk or in the car, then walking every day, gradually increasing the duration (up to 45 minutes) and intensity over the six weeks is a perfectly reasonable fitness goal. If you are already active, aim to move most of your exercise outdoors during this six weeks. As you become more accustomed to Ice Living, dip into the exercise chapter and try new activities to boost your calorie burning.

DAY 1

Meal 1 Breakfast/Brunch: Glass of cold water and lemon followed by Proper Porridge topped with sliced mango and kiwi fruit.

Meal 2 Lunch: Spicy Broccoli Salad. Add a slice of rye or granary seeded bread if needed.

Meal 3 Dinner: Chicken breast baked with garlic and lemon zest/juice, served with large green salad, roasted nuts and seeds.

Did you know? Chicory leaves make a great salad bowl addition as they are packed with a soluble fibre called inulin which helps to promote good bowel habits. It's also known to be an effective prebiotic, enabling the gut to hold on to the beneficial bacteria it needs to stay healthy.

Activity Kick off your new regimen with a gentle 15-minute walk outside. Walking is a great start to any fitness programme and yet it's often overlooked in favour of expensive gym classes. Despite recommendations that we should amass at least 10,000–12,000 steps a day through walking just to stay healthy – and even more (up to 15,000) to lose weight – most people manage just 3,000–4,000 a day.

Cooling strategy Decrease use of non-essential heating – that's heated towel rails, under-floor heating, heated seats in cars and extra home radiators.

DAY 2

Meal 1 Breakfast/Brunch: Glass of cold water and lemon followed by a bowl of low-fat Greek yoghurt piled with berries and served with a slice of rye or granary seeded bread/toast and cream cheese.

Meal 2 Lunch: Ceviche of Monkfish.

Meal 3 Dinner: Coconut Vegetable Curry with brown rice.

Did you know? Strawberries are more than just a great source of vitamin C and fibre. Plant chemicals called p-coumaric acid and chlorogenic acid that are present in the fruit can help to prevent the formation of carcinogenic (cancer-forming) substances called nitrosamines in the stomach, thereby lowering the risk of stomach cancer if you eat them regularly.

Activity Walk 5 minutes at a steady pace; walk briskly for 20 seconds, then at a steady pace for 20 seconds and then fast for 20 seconds – repeat the sequence 5 times; finally, walk 5 minutes at a moderate pace.

Cooling strategy Get into the habit of carrying extra layers and putting them on rather than vice versa, when you go outside. Carry extra clothing, but don't wear it unless you absolutely need it.

DAY 3

Meal 1 Breakfast/Brunch: Glass of cold water and lemon followed by Blueberry Omelette.

Meal 2 Lunch: Veggie-stuffed Pitta.

Meal 3 Dinner: Portuguese-style Chicken served with leafy green vegetables including kale and spinach.

Did you know? Blueberries are another fruit that are great for piling on porridge, yoghurt and muesli at breakfast time. Their countless health benefits are linked to the high levels of flavonoids they contain. These active substances include anthocyanin, the pigment that gives the berry its blue colour. Diets supplemented with blueberries have been shown to help prevent age-associated memory loss and boost brainpower. Research has also highlighted the cholesterol-fighting benefits of another blueberry ingredient, pterostilbene.

Activity Walk 20 minutes at a steady pace.

Cooling strategy Open a window in the room you are sitting or working in. In winter have it open for at least 5 minutes every hour.

DAY 4

Meal 1 Breakfast/Brunch: Glass of cold water and lemon followed by a bowl of Overnight Muesli (there should be enough for tomorrow as well).

Meal 2 Lunch: Watercress Soup with one or two slices of rye or granary seeded/multigrain bread.

Meal 3 Dinner: Carrot Veggie Burgers served with green salad and granary roll.

Did you know? Carrots are rich in beta carotene, the substance that gives them their vibrant orange colour. They are also packed with powerful antioxidants. However, they are better for you lightly cooked than completely raw and studies show that the anti-cancer properties are more potent if the vegetable is not cut up before cooking. Scientists found that cooked-before-cut carrots contained up to 35 per cent more of the beneficial compounds as chopped and grated carrot.

Activity Walk 5 minutes at a steady pace then 5 minutes at a brisk pace, and repeat.

Cooling strategy Reduce heating in the bedroom by a notch on the dial or by 1 °C.

DAY 5

Meal 1 Breakfast/Brunch: Glass of cold water with lemon followed by Overnight Muesli.

Meal 2 Lunch: Salad Niçoise.

Meal 3 Dinner: Spicy Chops served with steamed seasonal vegetables.

Did you know? Avoid buying ready-bagged salads. In non-organic produce, the manufacturing techniques used to keep the bagged greens crispy for longer have been shown to destroy vitamins and minerals as well as cells within the leaves. The process, called modified atmosphere packaging, is particularly damaging to vitamin C, one of the most important nutrients in salad leaves. In addition, pillows of leaves labelled as 'ready washed' can have been doused in water containing chemicals which can also affect nutrient levels.

Activity Take stairs and steps wherever you find them. There are countless proven benefits. Climbing stairs and steps for an average of 6 minutes a day led to a 15 per cent drop in cholesterol and a 10–15 per cent increase in fitness after eight weeks, one study at the University of Ulster found. It is also among the best bottom- and leg-toning activities around. Taking stairs one at a time is better than bounding up them when it comes to weight loss. Scientists from the University of Roehampton found climbing five flights of stairs five times a week – an ascent of around fifteen metres – burned an average of 302 calories if the stairs were taken one at a time, but only 260 if two stairs were taken at a time.

Cooling strategy Take a cooler shower – if you usually turn up the temperature to its max, reduce by a few notches.

DAY 6

Meal 1 Breakfast/Brunch: Glass of cold water with lemon followed by Fancy Scrambled Eggs.

Meal 2 Lunch: Tomato and Red Pepper Soup with a slice of rye bread or granary roll.

Meal 3 Dinner: Salmon and Broccoli Noodles.

Did you know? Broccoli is a rich source of vitamins C and K – important for healthy blood clotting – but it also contains a substance called indole-3-carbinol that helps to balance oestrogen levels. A study at Oregon State University found that cruciferous vegetables, including broccoli, are also among the richest in compounds that fight cancer.

Activity Walk 10 minutes steady, 10 minutes fast, 10 minutes steady.

Cooling strategy Turn down the central heating in the main living area by a notch or by 1 °C. Put on an extra layer until you acclimatize.

DAY 7

Meal 1 Breakfast/Brunch: Glass of cold water with lemon followed by Wholemeal Pancakes served with a dessertspoon of low-fat Greek yoghurt, sliced banana and a handful of chopped and flaked nuts.

Meal 2 Lunch: Butternut Squash Salad.

Meal 3 Dinner: Fiery Prawn Stir-fry

Did you know? Almonds are a great nut to add to your diet as they are rich in magnesium and calcium. Researchers have shown that they can help to boost weight loss. When a group of women consumed 40 almonds a day, they gained no weight in a six-month trial. It seems that not all of the fat in almonds is absorbed by the body.

Activity A gentle 25-minute walk.

Cooling strategy Subject yourself to a cold blast. In winter this can be simply heading outside on a chilly day for 5 minutes. In summer, finish a shower with a cool blast of water for 20 seconds.

DAY 8

Meal 1 Breakfast/Brunch: Glass of cold water with lemon followed by a bowl of low-fat Greek yoghurt piled with berries.

Meal 2 Lunch: Watercress Soup served with a slice of rye or granary seeded bread.

Meal 3 Dinner: Thai Beef Salad.

Did you know? Watercress is a powerhouse leaf that has been linked to cancer prevention when eaten regularly. One serving provides a quarter of your daily vitamin C content. Scientists at Southampton University found that volunteers who ate 80g of watercress a day – a single portion – had elevated levels of cancer-fighting molecules.

Activity Walk 5 minutes steady, walk briskly for 1 minute, steady for 2 minutes and repeat four times. Finally, walk 5 minutes steady.

Cooling strategy Reduce the tog of your duvet and consider the clothes you wear (if any) to bed. Are those thick, fleecy pyjamas really necessary? Likewise, do you need that extra layer of bedding or the fleecy thermal sheets?

DAY 9

Meal 1 Breakfast/Brunch: Glass of cold water with lemon followed by Perfect Muesli.

Meal 2 Lunch: Tomato and Red Pepper Soup served with a slice of rye or granary seeded bread.

Meal 3 Dinner: Salmon Fishcakes with Asparagus served with one other seasonal vegetable.

Did you know? A team from Bristol University found that men who consumed more than ten portions of tomatoes each week – such as fresh tomatoes, tomato juice and tomato in soups and sauces – saw an 18 per cent reduction in prostate cancer risk. The fruit's cancer-fighting properties are thought to be due to lycopene, an antioxidant which can protect against DNA and cell damage and which is more potent when cooked.

Activity Walk 20 minutes at a brisk pace.

Cooling strategy Spend at least an hour of every day outside. Sounds a lot, but in reality that is only 5 minutes an hour.

DAY 10

Meal 1 Breakfast/Brunch: Glass of cold water with lemon followed by Proper Porridge topped with chopped apple (peel on).

Meal 2 Lunch: Russian Borscht with a slice of rye or granary seeded bread.

Meal 3 Dinner: Tangy Swordfish served with steamed seasonal vegetables.

Did you know? Not only do apples and their peel help to activate good fat, but there are plenty of other benefits that come from eating them. They contain phytonutrients (plant compounds) which act as antioxidants against 'bad' LDL cholesterol and are rich in pectins, also helpful in reducing cholesterol levels.

Activity Warm up, skip as fast as you can for 45 seconds, rest for 2 minutes and repeat. Cool down.

Cooling strategy If you are usually a gym-goer, aim to switch at least 50 per cent of your workouts to outdoors.

DAY 11

Meal 1 Breakfast/Brunch: Glass of cold water with lemon followed by Overnight Muesli.

Meal 2 Lunch: Watercress and Quinoa Salad.

Meal 3 Dinner: Vegetable Stir-fry with Cashews.

Did you know? Quinoa is a relatively new player in the cereal grain scene, but has risen sharply in popularity due to its excellent amino acid profile – it contains all nine essential amino acids, making it a complete protein source. It is among the least allergenic of all grains, making it a fantastic wheat-free choice. Quinoa contains small amounts of the healthy omega-3 fatty acids and in comparison to common cereals has a higher content of monounsaturated fat.

Activity Warm up with a gentle 5-minute walk, walk as fast as you can for 2 minutes, then cool down with a gentle 5-minute walk.

Cooling strategy Exercise wearing one less layer than usual. Ditch the base layer or gilet, shower-proof top when not raining or arm warmers (yes, really).

DAY 12

Meal 1 Breakfast/Brunch: Glass of cold water with lemon followed by Overnight Muesli.

Meal 2 Lunch: Stuffed Red Peppers.

Meal 3 Dinner: Fritatta Verdi served with a salad containing green leaves, tomatoes and seeds.

Did you know? Red peppers are another good source of the carotenoid pigment lycopene, which is a powerful antioxidant linked to a lower risk of prostate, pancreatic and cervical cancers. They are also rich in pigments called lutein and zeaxanthin, naturally found in the retina, consumption of which can help prevent macular degeneration, a condition that can impair the vision of older people.

Activity 30 minutes brisk walking.

Cooling strategy Take an ice-cold drink before a workout, not after it.

DAY 13

Meal 1 Breakfast/Brunch: Glass of cold water with lemon followed by Proper Muesli.

Meal 2 Lunch: Tuna Sandwich.

Meal 3 Dinner: Barley Chicken served with a steamed leafy green vegetable.

Did you know? Choose kale as a leafy green. A form of cabbage, it has more calcium than broccoli and is high in vitamins A and C. It's also a good source of iron and contains plenty of vitamin K and the pigment lutein, important for healthy vision. If curly kale is too tough and fibrous for your taste buds, try baby leaf kale which is quicker to cook and more tender.

Activity Find a patch of grass about 60–80 metres long in a park or football pitch. It can be gently sloping uphill or flat. Warm up for 5 minutes with a gentle walk and then walk fast over the distance (or up the slope), pumping your arms. Walk back at a moderate pace to recover. Repeat 4 times. Cool down for 5 minutes with a gentle walk.

Cooling strategy Give up (or cut down) on hot or Bikram yoga. Try yoga outdoors, or yoga-hiking.

DAY 14

Meal 1 Breakfast/Brunch: Glass of cold water with lemon followed by Blueberry Omelette.

Meal 2 Lunch: Ceviche of Monkfish.

Meal 3 Dinner: Coconut Vegetable Curry served with brown rice.

Did you know? Cooking without heat is a great way to embrace the Ice Diet principles. Jamie Oliver includes a chapter on the various techniques in his book *Jamie Oliver's Kitchen* (Penguin Books).

Activity Warm up, skip as fast as you can for 60 seconds, rest for 2 minutes and repeat. Cool down.

Cooling strategy Try a contrast shower. I started with 5×10-second bursts of cool water towards the end of the shower, building up to 10×10 seconds. It should not be torturous. Allow your body to adapt. You will probably find, as I did, that it leaves you more refreshed than a steaming hot blast.

DAY 15

Meal 1 Breakfast/Brunch: Glass of cold water with lemon followed by Fancy Scrambled Eggs.

Meal 2 Lunch: Broad Bean and Quinoa Salad.

Meal 3 Dinner: Portuguese-style Chicken served with lightly steamed seasonal vegetables.

Did you know? It's no coincidence that I find eggs the most satisfying of brunch options and that they keep me well and truly full until my second meal. US researchers described eggs as 'nature's appetite suppressant' after a study found that when people had scrambled eggs for breakfast they were less hungry at lunchtime than when they started the day with a processed breakfast cereal. Eggs' satiating effects are attributed to the high level of protein they contain. Levels of ghrelin, a hunger hormone, are found to be lower in breakfast egg eaters, while levels of PYY, a hormone that helps make us feel full, are higher.

Activity Walk or jog for 3 minutes at a moderate pace. Then 'sprint' walk for 20 seconds (at a speed that makes your thighs burn after 15 seconds). Revert to moderate pace for 2 minutes and repeat twice more (3×20-second sprints in total). Cool down.

Cooling strategy Get into the habit of opening a window an hour before you go to bed. By all means close it again before you head between the sheets until you get used to the cooler environment.

DAY 16

Meal 1 Breakfast/Brunch: Glass of cold water with lemon followed by Rhubarb Bircher.

Meal 2 Lunch: Salad Niçoise.

Meal 3 Dinner: Rice Pasta and Smoked Salmon.

Did you know? Rhubarb is a much-overlooked garden fruit that has potent health benefits. Researchers at Sheffield Hallam University found that cooking rhubarb for 20 minutes dramatically increases its levels of anti-cancer chemicals.

Activity Gentle 35-minute walk.

Cooling strategy Invest in workout gloves and a headband rather than thermal base layers; thermal socks rather than leggings.

DAY 17

Meal 1 Breakfast/Brunch: Glass of cold water with lemon followed by Poached Eggs with Avocado and Spinach.

Meal 2 Lunch: Spiced Apple and Rice.

Meal 3 Dinner: Thai Beef Salad.

Did you know? Avocados provide one of the highest amounts of protein of any fruit. They are also loaded with the mineral potassium, containing more than double the amount in a banana. Potassium is crucial for life and necessary for the heart, kidneys and other organs to work normally.

Activity Walk 5 minutes steady, 30 seconds fast, 30 seconds steady (repeat 6 times); walk 10 minutes steady.

Cooling strategy If you are a regular swimmer, test local pools to find the coolest. Some private pools alternate temperatures throughout the day. Swim when it's set at the cooler end of the thermal spectrum.

DAY 18

Meal 1 Breakfast/Brunch: Glass of cold water with lemon followed by Quinoa Fruit Salad.

Meal 2 Lunch: Watercress Soup served with a slice of rye or granary seeded bread.

Meal 3 Dinner: Salmon and Broccoli Noodles.

Did you know? Made with flour produced from the rye kernal, rye bread has a dark colour from the caramelization of the starch in the grain and a dense texture which makes it very filling. You will find one slice more than enough as an accompaniment to your lunch. Studies have shown that rye bread is great for staving off hunger pangs. It's also a low GI bread, meaning you get a more sustained release of energy.

Activity Warm up, skip as fast as you can for 90 seconds, cool down.

Cooling strategy Reduce heating in your home by another degree (remember the ultimate goal is 19 or 20 °C during the autum and winter months).

DAY 19

Meal 1 Breakfast/Brunch: Glass of cold water with lemon followed by Perfect Muesli.

Meal 2 Lunch: Veggie-stuffed Pitta with Feta Cheese.

Meal 3 Dinner: Spicy Chops served with steamed leafy green vegetables.

Did you know? Feta is a Greek cheese made with sheep's milk. It's tasty and tangy and, what's more, low in calories, containing only 85 per 30g serving. It is higher in sodium than some cheeses due to the fact that it's aged in salty brine, so not one to be eating every day. But a delicious addition to this Veggie-stuffed Pitta.

Activity Walk 45 minutes at a steady pace.

Cooling strategy Try a foot plunge pool. Celebrity trainer Jon Denoris recommends his clients fill a basin with ice-cold water and put their feet in for up to 15 minutes first thing in the morning.

DAY 20

Meal 1 Breakfast/Brunch: Glass of cold water with lemon followed by Coconut Pancakes served with low-fat Greek yoghurt and berries.

Meal 2 Lunch: Russian Borscht with a slice of rye or granary seeded bread.

Meal 3 Dinner: Carrot Veggie Burger in a granary bun served with a large green salad, a glug of olive oil and seeds.

Did you know? Beetroot contains compounds called nitrates that have been repeatedly shown in studies to aid recovery time and sports performance. It could have other benefits, including boosting cognitive power. When you eat high-nitrate foods, good bacteria in the mouth turn nitrate into nitrite. Research has found that nitrites can help open up the blood vessels in the body, increasing blood flow and oxygen specifically to places that are lacking oxygen, including the brain.

Activity Find a patch of grass about 60–80 metres long in a park or football pitch. It can be gently sloping uphill or flat. Warm up for 5 minutes with a gentle walk and then walk fast over the distance (or up the slope), pumping your arms. Walk back at a moderate pace back to recover. Repeat 6 times. Cool down for 5 minutes with a gentle walk.

Cooling strategy Take a cooler bath. I used to find I knelt in my bath for 5 minutes or more because it was just too hot to lie down. Not any more – a cooler bath is not only healthier, but more pleasurable.

DAY 21

Meal 1 Breakfast/Brunch: Glass of cold water with lemon followed by Wholemeal Pancakes served with low-fat Greek yoghurt and halved cherries.

Meal 2 Lunch: Spicy Broccoli Salad.

Meal 3 Dinner: Tangy Swordfish with steamed seasonal vegetables.

Did you know? Cherries are rich in D-gluaric acid, a super-nutrient said to help lower cholesterol. With an exceptionally low GI, they are also great for stabilizing blood sugar levels and keeping hunger at bay. They contain good levels of potassium, which regulates heart function, as well as a cancer-protecting substance called ellegic acid.

Activity Gentle 20-minute stroll.

Cooling strategy Check that the temperature of your workplace is within healthy limits. As low as 16 °C is considered 'reasonable' in the UK. If 10–15 per cent of your colleagues feel the environment is too stuffy, you have a case to push for change.

DAY 22

Meal 1 Breakfast/Brunch: Glass of cold water with lemon followed by scrambled eggs (made with 2 free-range, organic eggs) and a slice of smoked salmon, chopped.

Meal 2 Lunch: Watercress and Quinoa Salad.

Meal 3 Dinner: Spring Seasonal Risotto.

Did you know? Asparagus is in season for just eight weeks from the end of April in the UK, so grab it for your seasonal risotto while you can. Each spear contains just 4 calories and half of that comes in the form of protein. Seven small spears constitute one serving.

Activity Walk 10 minutes steady, 8 minutes at a brisk pace, 3 minutes at a fast pace, then 4 minutes steady.

Cooling strategy Reduce heating in the bedroom by another notch.

DAY 23

Meal 1 Breakfast/Brunch: Glass of cold water with lemon followed by Rhubarb Bircher.

Meal 2 Lunch: Tomato and Red Pepper Soup served with a slice of rye or granary seeded bread.

Meal 3 Dinner: Spicy Chops served with fresh beans or peas and a steamed cruciferous vegetable – sprouts, broccoli and cauliflower are the best choices.

Did you know? Cruciferous vegetables contain potent cancer-fighting properties. Those who ate them at least weekly cut the risk of mouth cancer and breast cancer by almost a fifth and oesophageal cancer by more than a quarter. A particular nutrient in cruciferous vegetables, which also include watercress and radish, can kill cancer cells and gives potential for the production of new drugs.

Activity 30–45-minute walk with a 5-minute fast burst in the middle.

Cooling strategy Get outside on a cold day for 2 or 3 minutes without a coat.

DAY 24

Meal 1 Breakfast/Brunch: Glass of cold water with lemon followed by Poached Eggs with Avocado and Spinach.

Meal 2 Lunch: Spiced Apple and Rice.

Meal 3 Dinner: Barley Chicken with steamed vegetables.

Did you know? Spinach contains green leaf membrane substances called thylakoids that have been shown to reinforce the body's production of satiety hormones and suppress 'hedonic' hunger – eating for pleasure rather than physical need. Eaten regularly, it can help lead to better appetite control, healthier eating habits and increased weight loss.

Activity Warm up. Skip as fast as you can for 60 seconds, then skip gently for 60 seconds. Repeat 4 times. Cool down.

Cooling strategy During the day, try switching temperatures in your home from 20 °C to 16 °C every hour, just for ten minutes at a time.

DAY 25

Meal 1 Breakfast/Brunch: Glass of cold water with lemon followed by Quinoa Fruit Salad.

Meal 2 Lunch: Stuffed Red Peppers.

Meal 3 Dinner: Fiery Prawn Stir-fry.

Did you know? Add kiwi fruit to your Quinoa Fruit Salad and it could help to improve your mood. Researchers from the University of Otago in Christchurch, New Zealand, found that a group who were eating kiwi fruit daily experienced significantly less fatigue and depression than a group who were not eating kiwi. They also felt they had more energy. These changes appeared to be related to the optimizing of vitamin C intake with the kiwi fruit dose. Kiwi fruit are an exceptional source of vitamin C.

Activity 30-minute brisk walk.

Cooling strategy Open a window at night when the weather outside is not freezing.

DAY 26

Meal 1 Breakfast/Brunch: Glass of cold water with lemon followed by Proper Porridge topped with dried or fresh figs or prunes, chopped.

Meal 2 Lunch: Tuna Sandwich.

Meal 3 Dinner: Salmon and Broccoli Noodles.

Did you know? Dried fruits are often maligned as being too concentrated in sugar to be healthy. And while they should not be consumed in excessive amounts for this reason, they have more than enough health benefits to warrant their addition to your morning porridge. Take prunes, which were shown in research at the University of Liverpool to aid weight control, not cause weight gain. Research at the University's Institute of Psychology, Health and Society tested whether eating prunes as part of a weight-loss diet helped or hindered weight control over a twelve-week period. Those who ate prunes every day (140g a day for women and 171g a day for men) lost 2kg in weight and shed 2.5cm off their waists compared to only 1.5kg in weight and 1.7cm from their waists among those given only 'healthy eating advice'.

Activity Walk or jog for 3 minutes at a moderate pace. Then 'sprint' walk for 20 seconds (at a speed that makes your thighs burn after 15 seconds). Revert to moderate pace for 2 minutes and repeat 4 times more (5×20-second sprints in total). Cool down.

Cooling strategy On warm nights (spring and autumn), reduce to a minimum tog rating with your duvet. Or try sleeping with just a sheet.

DAY 27

Meal 1 Breakfast/Brunch: Glass of cold water with lemon followed by a bowl of fresh fruit salad made with a variety of fruits. Choose from: berries, apple, pear, kiwi, mango, pineapple. Top with a spoonful of plain yoghurt and some seeds.

Meal 2 Lunch: Veggie-stuffed Pitta with Feta Cheese.

Meal 3 Dinner: Rice Pasta with Smoked Salmon.

Did you know? Eating apples and pears regularly may boost your protection against strokes. A Dutch study found that eating 'white-coloured' fruit and vegetables was associated with a 52 per cent lower stroke risk – and apples and pears were the main foods consumed in the study.

Activity Walk easy for 5 minutes, fast for 2 minutes, easy for 5 minutes, fast for 2 minutes, easy for 5 minutes.

Cooling strategy Increase your time spent outside to a minimum of 90 minutes a day (an average of 7–8 minutes an hour).

DAY 28

Meal 1 Breakfast/Brunch: Glass of cold water with lemon followed by Overnight Muesli.

Meal 2 Lunch: Watercress Soup served with a slice of rye or granary seeded bread.

Meal 3 Dinner: Thai Beef Salad.

Did you know? Oats are among the only cereal grains to contain a particular fibre called beta-glucan, which has been found to lower cholesterol and so help to protect against heart disease. Oats have also been linked to lower blood pressure. They are a source of folic acid, which is essential for healthy foetal development, and also contain vitamin B1 (thiamin), which is crucial for the nervous system.

Activity 45-minute walk or cycle.

Cooling strategy Reduce the amount of time and the temperature of car heating on cold days. Practise the 'blast' approach with warm and then cold air.

DAY 29

Meal 1 Breakfast/Brunch: Glass of cold water with lemon followed by Overnight Muesli.

Meal 2 Lunch: Watercress and Quinoa Salad.

Meal 3 Dinner: Coconut Vegetable Curry served with brown rice.

Did you know? Proof that over-cooking vegetables diminishes their nutrient content came in the form of a study at the University of

Warwick. Researchers there found that boiling brassica vegetables such as broccoli, Brussel sprouts, cauliflower and green cabbage for too long (30 minutes) had a serious impact on the retention of important glucosinolate, cancer-preventing substances, with levels dropping by up to 77 per cent.

Activity Warm up. Run, walk or cycle hard (but not flat out) for 60 seconds. Run, walk or cycle at a gentle pace for 90 seconds to recover. Repeat 4 times. Cool down.

Cooling strategy If you feel 'cold' indoors, step outside and walk around briskly, skip or jog for 5 minutes to re-set your temperature gauge.

DAY 30

Meal 1 Breakfast/Brunch: Glass of cold water with lemon followed by Coconut Pancakes served with a dessertspoon of low-fat Greek yoghurt and berries.

Meal 2 Lunch: Tomato and Red Pepper Soup served with a slice of rye or granary seeded bread.

Meal 3 Dinner: Tangy Swordfish with a small baked sweet potato and a large green salad with seeds.

Did you know? Unlike coconut water (found inside the fleshy meat), the coconut milk used in these pancakes is made by grating the white coconut flesh and soaking it in hot water, which sees the coconut cream rise to the top so that it can be skimmed off. The remaining liquid is squeezed to extract what we know as coconut milk. Coconuts are rich in a range of vitamins and minerals including C, E, the B group, iron, selenium and magnesium. The milk is relatively high in fat, but mostly the beneficial variety of medium-chain fatty acids such as lauric acid, which is converted by the body into an antiviral and antibacterial compound called manolaurin, said to protect against illness.

Activity 45-minute walk or cycle.

Cooling strategy Try outdoor swimming. It is the perfect accompaniment to the Ice Diet. If you haven't ventured into outside waters before, then lidos are the perfect starting point.

DAY 31

Meal 1 Breakfast/Brunch: Glass of cold water with lemon followed by Fancy Scrambled Eggs.

Meal 2 Lunch: Butternut Squash Salad.

Meal 3 Dinner: Vegetable Stir-fry with Cashews.

Did you know? The orange-yellow colour of butternut squash comes from the high levels of beta carotene it contains. In the body, beta carotene is converted to vitamin A, a fat-soluble vitamin which helps maintain eye health, healthy mucous membranes and other soft tissues. It also plays a role in promoting healthy skin.

Activity Walk 5 minutes steady, walk briskly for 1 minute, steady for 2 minutes then repeat 6 times. Walk 5 minutes steady.

Cooling strategy Reduce heating by another degree to edge closer to the optimum 18 or 19 °C. Remember not to go lower than this, apart from an occasional cold blast.

DAY 32

Meal 1 Breakfast/Brunch: Glass of cold water with lemon followed by Rhubarb Bircher.

Meal 2 Lunch: Spicy Broccoli Salad.

Meal 3 Dinner: Barley Chicken served with a leafy green vegetable, steamed.

Did you know? Cinnamon is another great spice to include in your Ice Diet and adds to the flavour of your Rhubarb Bircher. The spice can inhibit the growth of the E. coli bacteria when added to foods and it might also help to lower blood sugar levels in people with Type 2 diabetes when consumed regularly.

Activity 30-minute hilly walk or cycle.

Cooling strategy Open a window when driving, even if it's for just a few minutes on a cold day.

DAY 33

Meal 1 Breakfast/Brunch: Glass of cold water with lemon followed by Proper Porridge topped with seeds and chopped nuts.

Meal 2 Lunch: Broad Bean and Quinoa Salad.

Meal 3 Dinner: Spicy Chops with seasonal vegetables, steamed.

Did you know? Broad beans are rich in both folate and B vitamins, which we need for nerve and blood-cell development, cognitive function and energy. Adding beans to a dish is also a way of lowering the GI content of the meal, meaning energy will be released slowly into the body, keeping you satisfied for longer.

Activity Walk or jog for 3 minutes at a moderate pace. Then 'sprint' walk for 20 seconds (at a speed that makes your thighs burn after 15 seconds). Revert to moderate pace for 2 minutes and repeat 4 times more (5×20-second sprints in total). Cool down.

Cooling strategy Embrace the seasons. Think about what you are wearing indoors and if it doesn't tally with the outdoor temperatures, then the likelihood is your home is too hot.

DAY 34

Meal 1 Breakfast/Brunch: Glass of cold water with lemon followed by Blueberry Pancakes with other berries added.

Meal 2 Lunch: Ceviche of Monkfish.

Meal 3 Dinner: Carrot Veggie Burgers served with a granary roll, tomato slices and a green salad.

Did you know? Blackcurrants are a good addition to your blueberry pancakes as they contain four times the vitamin C in an orange. The skins of the fruit contain anthocyanin, which is known to inhibit bacteria – a common cause of stomach complaints.

Activity 10 minutes easy run, walk or cycle followed by 4×30-second 'sprints' (each followed by a 60-second recovery). Finally, 10 minutes at easy pace.

Cooling strategy When you wash up, do so with cooler water than normal. Remember that exposing your hands to cold and cool water is a highly effective way to boost good fat activity.

DAY 35

Meal 1 Breakfast/Brunch: Glass of cold water with lemon followed by bowl of fresh fruit salad made with a variety of fruits. Choose from: berries, apple, pear, kiwi, mango, pineapple. Top with a spoonful of plain yoghurt and some chopped walnuts.

Meal 2 Lunch: Stuffed Red Peppers.

Meal 3 Dinner: Salmon Fishcakes with Asparagus and one other seasonal vegetable, steamed.

Did you know? Walnuts contain high levels of manganese and copper as well as an antioxidant compound called ellagic acid – this helps to block metabolic processes that trigger the inflammation that can lead to insulin resistance and diabetes. Regularly eating walnuts has also been shown to reduce cholesterol levels.

Activity 45-minute walk or cycle with a 10-minute 'fast section' in the middle.

Cooling strategy Drink icy cool water. It might not have a significant effect on calorie burning, but it does help to prepare body and mind for cooling.

DAY 36

Meal 1 Breakfast/Brunch: Glass of cold water with lemon followed by Poached Egg with Avocado and Spinach.

Meal 2 Lunch: Spiced Apple and Rice.

Meal 3 Dinner: Frittata Verdi served with a large green salad, roasted walnuts, olive oil and 30g of crumbled feta cheese.

Did you know? There's nothing better than a perfectly cooked yellow egg yolk to tempt your appetite. And they're nutritionally beneficial as well as tasting delicious. Egg yolks contain the nutrients lutein and zeax-anthin, which have been shown to prevent or even help to reverse the age-related eye problem macular degeneration. Since spinach is also a great supplier of lutein, this is a super-healthy dish as far as your vision is concerned.

Activity Find a patch of grass about 60–80 metres long in a park or football pitch. It can be gently sloping uphill or flat. Warm up for 5 minutes with a gentle walk and then walk or run fast over the distance (or up the slope), pumping your arms. Walk at a moderate pace back to recover. Repeat 8 times. Cool down for 5 minutes with a gentle walk or jog.

Cooling strategy Try ice skating, one of the few sports that is cool indoors as well as out. Indoor ski slopes are another option.

DAY 37

Meal 1 Breakfast/Brunch: Glass of cold water with lemon followed by Quinoa Fruit Salad.

Meal 2 Lunch: Large sweet potato, baked and served with a dollop of crème fraîche or low-fat Greek yoghurt and sprinkled with freshly cut herbs.

Meal 3 Dinner: Spicy Prawn Stir-fry.

Did you know? Sweet potatoes get their bright orange colour from beta carotene, of which they are an abundant source. But that's not all. When US scientists compiled tables of 58 vegetables ranked according to their content of 7 important nutrients, sweet potatoes scored 582 compared with a paltry 114 from ordinary spuds.

Activity 30-minute walk.

Cooling strategy Get up for an early-morning 'frost' walk when the cool mornings set in. There is no better time of the day to experience cool living.

DAY 38

Meal 1 Breakfast/Brunch: Glass of cold water with lemon followed by Proper Porridge topped with grated apple and chopped walnuts.

Meal 2 Lunch: Russian Borscht with a slice of rye or granary seeded bread.

Meal 3 Dinner: Portuguese-style Chicken with two or three seasonal vegetables, steamed.

Did you know? Porridge is hailed as one of the healthiest breakfasts and brunches around because of the combination of fibre, vitamins and minerals it contains. But there's growing evidence that a bio-active compound, only contained in oats, may possess antioxidant properties, which help it to protect against both cancer and heart problems. And researchers think that the compound, called avenanthramide, could stop fat forming in the arteries, a cause of heart attacks and strokes.

Activity Walk 5 minutes steady, walk briskly for 1 minute, steady for 2 minutes and repeat 8 times. Finally, walk 5 minutes steady.

Cooling strategy Try a night-time cooling shower a few minutes before heading to bed. It can have the added effect of boosting melatonin production, enhancing sleep.

DAY 39

Meal 1 Breakfast/Brunch: Glass of cold water with lemon followed by Fancy Scrambled Eggs.

Meal 2 Lunch: Broad Bean and Quinoa Salad.

Meal 3 Dinner: Coconut Vegetable Curry served with brown rice.

Did you know? An egg yolk contains thirteen essential nutrients, including the B-vitamin group which is needed for vital functions in the body. Egg whites contain albumen which is an important source of protein but not fat.

Activity Warm up. Run, walk or cycle hard (but not flat out as for the shorter sprints) for 40 seconds. Run, walk or cycle at a gentle pace for 90 seconds to recover. Repeat 8 times. Cool down.

Cooling strategy Reduce bedroom heat by another notch, aiming for the optimal 19 to 20 °C.

DAY 40

Meal 1 Breakfast/Brunch: Glass of cold water with lemon followed by Wholemeal Pancakes stuffed with one dessertspoon of low-fat Greek yoghurt, a sliced banana and seeds.

Meal 2 Lunch: Tomato and Red Pepper Soup.

Meal 3 Dinner: Seasonal Spring Risotto.

Did you know? Seeds are one of my favourite ingredients to add to any breakfast-in-a-dish. Among the best are roasted pumpkins seeds, rich in the amino acids alanin, glycene and glutamic acid; seasame seeds, which are a well-known source of vitamin E plus omega-6 and monounsaturated fats; and sunflower seeds, rich in the B-complex vitamins, which are essential for a healthy nervous system, and are a good source of phosphorus, magnesium, iron, calcium, potassium, protein and vitamin E.

Activity 20-minute brisk walk.

Cooling strategy Aim to spend a total of 2 hours a day outside – that equates to just 10 minutes for every waking hour.

DAY 41

Meal 1 Breakfast/Brunch: Glass of cold water with lemon followed by Perfect Muesli.

Meal 2 Lunch: Salad Niçoise.

Meal 3 Dinner: Salmon Fishcakes served with a large green salad, tomatoes, peppers, olive oil and roasted cashews.

Did you know? Cashews are packed with iron, containing double the amount of many other nuts and twice the concentration you will find in minced beef. Just 25 cashew nuts a day provide the level of iron needed by an adult woman.

Cooling strategy Maintain a 19 to 20 °C temperature at home most of the time.

DAY 42

Meal 1 Breakfast/Brunch: Glass of cold water with lemon followed by Blueberry Pancakes.

Meal 2 Lunch: Spicy Broccoli Salad.

Meal 3 Dinner: Portuguese-style Chicken with two seasonal vegetables, steamed.

Did you know? Ginger has many health benefits including aiding circulation. But studies have shown that, eaten regularly, it can also reduce exercise-induced muscle soreness by as much as 25 per cent.

Activity Walk, cycle or jog for 5 minutes at a moderate pace. Then 'sprint' for 20 seconds (at a speed that makes your thighs burn after 15 seconds). Revert to moderate pace for 2 minutes and repeat 5 times more (6×20-second sprints in total). Cool down.

Cooling strategy Keep cool. Ensure the changes you have made are implemented long term. Check in with your family regularly to make sure they are comfortable with the living temperature at home, but the likelihood is that they will barely notice the changes as they have been carried out so gradually.

Ice Diet Maintenance

After six weeks on the Ice Diet plan you will almost certainly have shed weight, gained lean muscle tissue (if you have increased your activity levels as recommended) and feel as well as look healthier. So what next? Given that this is a plan for life, the idea is to keep up the good work. As you will have discovered, this is no starvation diet. It is wholesome and nutrient dense, almost completely depleted of unnecessary processed and refined foods. When it comes to meal schedules, try to stick within the 'window' that most suits your lifestyle and work commitments. Once you've reached your target weight, there are grounds for adopting a more flexible approach. Among friends who have tested the plan, many choose to eat two meals on three days and three meals the rest of the week. The important things are to stay within your eating 'window' and to avoid snacking whenever possible. Cooling strategies, of course, are for life. And by now the likelihood is that you will barely register how much cooler your life has become. Only when you enter rooms and environments out of your control, with Saharan levels of heat, will you appreciate just how far you have come for the good of your health.

8 Ice Diet Recipes

All of the recipes on the Ice Diet are interchangeable. By that, I mean they can be eaten at any time of the day as long as you stick to your two or three meal total. For ease of navigation I have grouped them as breakfast/brunch, lunch or dinner recipes. The breakfast/brunch recipes are lighter and the dinner recipes more substantial. But if you prefer to have an omelette for your evening meal rather than lunch, for example, then just switch accordingly. Serving portions are listed with each recipe. If a recipe serves 2–4, feel free to make it a slightly larger portion if needed, but not to eat the whole thing on your own. Listen to your body and learn to stop when you have had enough. The important thing is to keep to your number of meals (no snacking!) and to eat within your meal schedule window.

Shopping List

This is by no means an exhaustive shopping list, more a helpful guide to the kind of store-cupboard essentials you will need to stock up on in order to get started.

Cinnamon

Cumin seeds

Sea salt

Black pepper

Turmeric

Chilli powder

Dijon mustard

Rapeseed oil

Olive oil

Sultanas

Nuts: hazelnuts, walnuts,
   cashews, almonds

Flaked almonds

Dried coconut

Desiccated coconut (unsweetened)

Porridge oats, rolled

Pinhead oatmeal

Medium oatmeal

Wholemeal flour

Flaked bran

Rye flakes

Rye bread

Vegetable-based or rice pasta

Dried organic apricots

Dried organic figs

Dried cranberries

Seeds: pumpkin, sesame,
   sunflower, etc.

Quinoa

Chickpeas

Butterbeans

Barley

Puy lentils

Wild rice

Chipotle paste

Balsamic vinegar

Runny honey

Anchovies

Tinned tuna

Rice noodles

Capers

Light soy sauce

Tomato puree

Peanut butter

Coconut milk (canned)

Vegetable or chicken stock

Risotto rice

Feta cheese

Low-fat Greek yoghurt

Low-fat crème fraîche

Breakfast/Brunch Recipes

Blueberry Omelette (serves 1)

1 large egg
1 tbsp milk
¼ tsp cinnamon
½ tsp rapeseed oil
100g cottage or low-fat cream cheese
175g blueberries (other berries can be added if you prefer)

Beat the egg, milk and cinnamon together. Heat oil in a frying pan and pour in the egg mixture to evenly cover the base. Cook for a few minutes until set and golden underneath. Pull egg from the edges to ensure it is thoroughly cooked through. Place on a plate, spoon over the cheese, then scatter with berries. Roll up and serve.

Overnight Muesli (serves 2–4)

This is one of my all-time favourite, filling brunch recipes. It keeps well in the fridge for a couple of days.

100g porridge oats
2 tbsp sultanas
300ml freshly squeezed orange juice
2 grated eating apples
milk (to mix)
nuts and seeds
berries

Put the oats, sultanas and orange juice in a mixing bowl. Cover and leave to soak overnight. Next morning, stir in the apple and milk to give a soft consistency. Spoon into dishes and top with chopped nuts, seeds and berries.

Proper Porridge (serves 1)

This is something of an extravagant take on porridge, but well worth the effort. It gets the thumbs-up from my Scottish partner.

25g pinhead oatmeal
25g medium oatmeal
100ml milk
200ml water
pinch of salt
splash of cold milk

Toast the oats in a dry frying pan for a few minutes. Then place them in a small saucepan along with the milk and water. Bring slowly to the boil, stirring frequently with a wooden spoon. Turn down the heat and simmer, stirring very regularly, for about 10 minutes, until you have the consistency you require. After about 5 minutes, add the salt. Cover and allow to sit for 5 minutes, then serve with a splash of cold milk and toppings of your choice. My favourites are chopped dried dates, grated apple (with skin) and chopped nuts.

Fancy Scrambled Eggs (serves 2)

½ tbsp butter
4 asparagus stalks
4 eggs
1 tbsp milk
50g smoked salmon
50g fresh goat's cheese, crumbled
black pepper

Heat the butter in a non-stick pan over a medium heat. When the butter begins to foam, add the asparagus and cook until just tender. Crack the eggs into a bowl and whisk with the milk. Season with black pepper and add to the pan with the asparagus. Turn the heat down to low and use a wooden spoon to constantly stir and scrape the eggs until they begin to 'curdle'. Just before they're done and while still liquidy, stir in the goat's cheese. Remove from the heat when the eggs are still creamy and soft, and fold in the chopped smoked salmon.

Wholemeal Pancakes (serves 2–4)

100–125g wholemeal flour
pinch of salt
1 egg
300ml (½ pint) milk
1 tsp rapeseed oil, plus a little extra for frying

Put the flour and salt in a bowl. Using a balloon whisk, beat the egg in a jug with the milk and oil, then pour this into the flour and whisk in until the batter is smooth. Let the batter stand for 20 minutes if you have time. Heat a little oil in a pancake pan and, when hot, pour in about 2 tbsp of the batter. Tilt the pan so the batter coats the base of the pan evenly. Cook for 2 to 3 minutes, then loosen the edge and flip the pancake over to cook the other side for 1 minute. Keep the cooked pancakes warm while you make more. They are perfect served with sweet or savoury fillings. Try low-fat Greek yoghurt with bananas and nuts.

Perfect Muesli (4–6 servings)

200g porridge oats

25g flaked bran

75g rye flakes

50g hazelnuts, lightly chopped

50g flaked almonds

50g sultanas

50g organic dried apricots

50g dried figs

2 tbsp pumpkin seeds

3 tsp sesame seeds

Preheat the oven to 160 °C/Gas 3. Place the oats, flaked bran, rye flakes, hazelnuts and almonds on a large baking tray and toast in the oven for 10 minutes, shaking and turning halfway through. Take the tray from the oven and leave to cool for about 10 minutes. Mix the toasted ingredients with everything else. Add other dried fruits if you prefer – apple, mango, dates or cherries. Serve with milk and top with fresh fruit. The remainder will keep in an airtight container.

Rhubarb Bircher (serves 2)

200g rhubarb cut into inch-long pieces
3 tbsp runny honey
120ml freshly squeezed orange juice
2 tbsp milk
120g rolled oats
1 tsp ground cinnamon
200g low-fat Greek yoghurt
50g toasted flaked almonds
50g toasted chopped hazelnuts

Place the rhubarb in a saucepan with the honey and orange juice and cook gently over a low heat for approximately 20 minutes until the rhubarb is slightly soft. Cool and drain the cooking liquid into a jug and add the milk to it. Mix the liquid with the oats, cinnamon, yoghurt, half the almonds and hazelnuts and half the rhubarb. Stir to combine and refrigerate overnight. Serve the muesli topped with the remaining poached rhubarb and nuts.

Poached Eggs with Avocado and Spinach (serves 2–4)

1 ripe medium avocado
4 cooked baby beetroot, quartered
handful of baby leaf spinach
drizzle of extra-virgin olive oil
small handful of toasted hazelnuts, roughly chopped
squeeze of lemon juice
4 large free-range eggs

Peel, stone and slice the avocado, then place in a bowl with the beetroot, spinach, olive oil, hazelnuts and lemon juice. Season and set aside. Poach the eggs: heat a large pan of salted water until it boils gently. Crack an egg into a small dish, then slide the egg into the water, lowering the dish as close to the water as possible. Repeat with the other eggs. Cook for 2–3 minutes, then remove with a slotted spoon and put the spoon on absorbent kitchen paper to dry the eggs. Divide the avocado mixture between however many servings, then put the eggs on top.

Quinoa Fruit Salad (serves 2–4)

170g quinoa
240ml water
pinch of salt
juice of 1 large lime
3 tbsp honey
2 tbsp finely chopped fresh mint

75g each of blueberries, blackberries, chopped
fresh pineapple, chopped kiwi fruit

Using a colander, rinse the quinoa under cold water. Add quinoa, water and salt to a medium saucepan and bring to the boil over medium heat. Boil for 5 minutes. Turn the heat to low and simmer for about 15 minutes, or until water is absorbed. Remove from heat and fluff with a fork. Let quinoa cool to room temperature. In a bowl, whisk the lime juice, honey and mint together until combined. In a separate bowl, combine quinoa, blueberries, blackberries, kiwi and pineapple. Pour honey-lime dressing over the fruit salad and mix until well combined. Garnish with additional mint, if desired. Serve at room temperature or chilled. You can add any combination of fresh fruit to this salad. Strawberries and mangoes are another good addition.

Coconut Pancakes (serves 2)

Being a long-time coconut fan, this is one of my favourite brunch recipes. It's also one of the easiest to make and is ultra-healthy – it will fill you up until the next mealtime.

3 medium free-range eggs
3 tbsp butter (melted) or coconut oil
3 tbsp coconut milk
1½ tsp honey
pinch of salt
3 tbsp coconut flour (available at health food stores)
½ tsp baking powder
a little extra butter for cooking

Whisk everything together well in a large jug. Heat a frying pan containing a little butter and pour in some of the mixture. Tilt the pan to the sides to ensure the mixture is evenly spread. Serve with low-fat Greek yoghurt and berries.

Lunch Recipes

Butternut Squash Salad (serves 2–4)

750g butternut squash, peeled and diced into 2cm cubes
glug of olive oil
15ml pure maple syrup
seasoning
3 tbsp dried cranberries
180ml apple juice
30ml cider vinegar
2 tbsp minced shallots
2 tsp Dijon mustard
125g rocket leaves
50g walnuts halves, toasted
75g freshly grated Parmesan

Preheat the oven to 200 °C/Gas 6. Put the butternut squash on a baking sheet, adding 2 tbsp olive oil, the maple syrup and seasoning, then toss so that it's all coated. Roast the squash for 15 minutes, turning once. Add the cranberries to the baking sheet for the last 5 minutes. Mix together the apple juice, vinegar and shallots in a small saucepan and bring to a boil over medium heat. Cook for around 6 minutes, until the liquid has reduced. Remove from the heat, whisk in the mustard, olive oil and seasoning. Place the rocket in a large salad bowl and add the roasted squash mixture, the walnuts and the grated cheese. Spoon some of the dressing over the salad and toss well. Serve immediately.

Watercress and Quinoa Salad (serves 2–4)

175g quinoa
1 medium head broccoli, broken into florets
2 tbsp hazelnut oil
zest and juice of 1 lemon
seasoning
25g hazelnuts
100g watercress
250g cherry tomatoes, halved
100g feta cheese, crumbled

Rinse the quinoa and cook in boiling water for about 15 minutes or until just tender. In a separate pan of boiling water, cook the broccoli florets for two minutes. Drain the quinoa and broccoli in a colander and rinse in cold water. When cold, put in a bowl. Add the oil, lemon zest and juice and seasoning. Toast the hazelnuts under a medium grill and roughly chop. Chop the watercress and add to the quinoa along with the hazelnuts, tomatoes and feta cheese.

Spicy Broccoli Salad (serves 2–4)

2 tbsp olive oil
1 tsp cumin seeds
1 clove of garlic, thinly sliced
1–2 small red chillis, finely chopped
200g broccoli, cut into whole florets
200g cooked or tinned chickpeas
1 medium red onion, sliced
1 medium red pepper, cut into matchsticks
2 tbsp lime juice
seasoning
handful of chopped coriander

Heat the oil in a wok or large frying pan and sauté the cumin seeds and garlic until the garlic is translucent. Add the red chilli and broccoli and sauté for another minute. Add the chickpeas, onion and red pepper. Sauté for 30 seconds and remove from heat. Add the lime juice and correct the seasoning with salt and pepper. Toss the coriander through and serve.

Veggie-stuffed Pitta with Feta Cheese (serves 2)

1½ tbsp balsamic vinegar
1½ tsp finely chopped fresh thyme
2 tsp Dijon mustard
2 tbsp olive oil
6–8 tbsp vegetable stock
3 tsp chopped basil
1 courgette, thinly sliced

8 small asparagus spears
1 red pepper, de-seeded and thinly sliced
2 wholemeal pitta breads
80g feta cheese

Make the marinade by whisking together the balsamic vinegar, fresh thyme, mustard, olive oil, stock and basil. Place the vegetables in a dish and pour the marinade on top. Leave for 25 minutes. Preheat a griddle and take the vegetables out of the marinade. Cook on the griddle for 2–3 minutes until just starting to brown. Toast the pitta, slice open and stuff with the vegetables and crumbled feta cheese before serving.

Broad Bean and Quinoa Salad (serves 2–4)

100g quinoa
700g broad beans, shelled
4 spring onions, chopped
2 tbsp extra-virgin olive oil
juice of 1 lemon
2 tbsp chopped mint or dill
100g watercress
150g feta, crumbled

Heat a frying pan to a medium heat. Add the quinoa and toast until it starts to pop. Transfer to a pan of boiling water. Simmer gently for around 15 minutes, until just tender. Boil the broad beans in another pan of simmering water for 3–4 minutes. Drain and cool in a bowl of cold water. Remove the tougher outer skins to reveal the vibrant green layer of bean beneath. Toss with the quinoa, spring onions, oil, lemon juice and mint or dill. Season. Serve on the watercress. Scatter over the feta.

Ceviche of Monkfish (serves 4–6)

This a great recipe that requires no cooking at all.

500g monkfish fillets
juice of 3 limes
1 medium hot red chilli, halved and seeded
1 small red onion
6 small tomatoes, skinned
3 tbsp olive oil
2 tbsp coriander
1 large, ripe avocado
seasoning

Cut the monkfish fillets into thin slices and place them in a shallow dish. Pour over the lime juice, making sure all of the fish pieces are covered. Place cling film over the dish and put in the fridge for 45 minutes. While the fish is cooling, slice the chillis finely and cut the onion into thin slices. Remove the seeds from the tomatoes and slice these finely too. Lift the monkfish out of the lime juice with a slotted spoon (the fish should be white and opaque by now) and place in a bowl with the chilli mixture. Add the coriander and olive oil and lightly toss all the ingredients together. Slice the avocado and place on serving dishes. Pile the ceviche mixture on top and serve.

Tomato and Red Pepper Soup (serves 4–6)

1 tbsp olive oil
1 onion, coarsely chopped
1 clove of garlic, chopped
3 red peppers, sliced
1 fresh red chilli, finely chopped
300ml chicken or vegetable stock
300ml sieved, cooked tomatoes
1 tbsp basil, chopped

Heat the oil in a saucepan over a low heat; stir in onion and garlic and cook gently until softened, about 5 minutes. Stir in the pepper slices and chopped chilli and cook for a further 5 minutes, stirring every now and again. Pour in the stock and remove from the heat. Puree the soup in a food processor or blender. Return the soup to the saucepan and stir in the sieved tomatoes. Season to taste and serve with chopped fresh basil leaves.

Quick Tuna Sandwich (serves 2)

1 160g can tuna in spring water, drained
1 small red onion
2 tomatoes, finely chopped
4 dashes Tabasco
4 tbsp low-fat cream or cottage cheese
4 slices granary seeded bread or rye bread

Mix together the tuna, onion, tomato and Tabasco in a bowl and season. Spread the cheese on two slices of the bread, top with the tuna mixture and the remaining slices of bread. Serve.

Stuffed Red Peppers (serves 2)

1 big red pepper or 2 smaller ones
½ mug of cooked brown rice
splash of olive oil
1 lemon, zest and juice
2 cloves of garlic, finely chopped
handful of almonds, sliced and toasted
handful of olives
pinch of chilli powder
100g feta cheese, crumbled
handful of herbs (mint, basil or parsley), chopped
handful of chopped dates
splash of cider vinegar
seasoning

Heat the oven to 200°C/Gas 6. Halve the pepper(s) lengthwise. Scrape seeds and pith out and put pepper(s) in a roasting tray. Add a splash of olive oil to the rice. Fold in the lemon zest, juice, garlic, almonds, olives, chilli powder, feta, herbs and dates. Add a splash of vinegar and season to taste. Divide the mix between the pepper halves. Drizzle olive oil over the top. Roast for 30 minutes and serve.

Salad Niçoise (serves 2)

300g small new potatoes
100g fine green beans, trimmed
3 organic, free-range eggs
5 tbsp olive oil
200g cherry tomatoes, halved
2 tbsp balsamic vinegar
handful of basil leaves
325g piece fresh tuna steak
juice ½ lemon
mix of lettuce and baby spinach leaves

For the Dressing:

50g black olives, pitted
5 marinated anchovies, fillets
1 clove of garlic
juice ½ lemon
4 tbsp olive oil
1 tbsp balsamic vinegar

To make the dressing, put the olives, anchovies and garlic into a bowl and mash with a pestle until you have a very rough paste. Stir in the lemon juice, olive oil and vinegar, then set aside. Cook the potatoes in boiling water for 12–15 minutes until tender, then drain and set aside. Cook the beans in boiling salted water for 4–5 minutes until tender. Drain, cool with cold water, then drain and set aside.

Boil water in a small pan and cook the eggs for 8–10 minutes. Halve the potatoes and heat 2 tbsp of oil in a non-stick frying pan. Place the potatoes cut-side down in the pan and sizzle for about 4 minutes until golden and crisp. Toss the potatoes in the pan to brown, then add the tomatoes. Fry the tomatoes for about 1 minute until just starting to blister, then season. Splash in 1 tbsp of the balsamic vinegar, then turn off the heat and scatter over the basil.

For the tuna, place a non-stick frying pan over a high heat, then turn the heat down and add 1 tbsp oil. Sear the tuna for 5 minutes without turning. Then turn over and repeat on the other side. Remove from the pan and allow the tuna to rest. To serve, whisk the remaining oil and vinegar with the lemon juice and toss in the leaves. Arrange the potatoes and tomatoes over, then put a pile of beans on top. Slice the tuna in half at a slight angle and place on top of the beans. Halve the eggs and add them to the top. Spoon the olive dressing over the eggs.

Spiced Apple and Rice (serves 2)

50g wild rice

50g long-grain brown rice

2 shallots, diced

½ sweet pointed Romano pepper or other red pepper,

deseeded and very finely sliced

1 celery stick, finely diced

1 apple, cored (not peeled) and diced

1 tomato, deseeded and finely diced

15g raisins

2 tbsp chopped fresh coriander
1/4 tsp chilli powder
2 tsp chipotle paste
2 tbsp low-fat Greek yoghurt

Bring a saucepan of water to the boil and add the rice. Gently simmer for 15–18 minutes until cooked. Drain in a colander and rinse in cold water. Drain again thoroughly and put into a large bowl. Add all the remaining ingredients and gently mix until combined. Season and serve.

Watercress Soup (serves 4)

1 litre chicken or vegetable stock
50g unsalted butter
250g watercress (3 good-sized bunches including stalks)
280g potatoes, peeled and finely sliced
seasoning
25g flat-leaf parsley, with stalks
1 tbsp crème fraîche

Bring the stock to the boil in a small saucepan. Melt the butter in a large saucepan over a medium heat, add the watercress and stir until it wilts. Add the potato slices and cook for a minute, then pour in the boiling stock and add some seasoning. Simmer the soup for six minutes, then liquidize in a blender with the parsley. Season to taste and serve with a dollop of crème fraîche.

Russian Borscht (serves 4–6)

This classic soup is thick and filling. Its rich colour is a giveaway that it is full of essential nutrients – beetroot is packed with vitamins, minerals and powerful antioxidants. Athletes consume beetroot juice to aid recovery. Prepared this way, it tastes delicious.

1kg small, fresh beetroot
50ml olive oil
1 large red onion, peeled and sliced
500g potatoes, peeled and diced
75g carrots
dash of Tabasco
3 cloves of garlic, peeled and chopped
seasoning
75ml vodka
juice of 1 lemon and 1 lime
1 tbsp low-fat Greek yoghurt and 1 tbsp dill for garnish

Wash and trim the beetroot and bring to the boil in a pan of water. Cook for 45 minutes until tender but not overly soft. Remove from the water but keep the water for later use. Remove the beetroot skins and chop the beetroot into quarters. Heat the oil and fry the onion until translucent, then add the diced potatoes, carrots, Tabasco, garlic and seasoning. Sauté for another 5 minutes. Add the beetroot and sauté for a further 2 minutes. Pour in the cooking liquid kept from earlier and simmer for 10 minutes. Add the vodka and lemon and lime juices. Take off the heat. Blend until smooth. Season to taste. Serve warm or chilled, with a dollop of low-fat Greek yoghurt and a sprinkling of chopped dill.

Dinner Recipes

Fiery Prawn Stir-fry (serves 4)

100g dried egg noodles
100g Tenderstem broccoli
2 tbsp olive oil
1 apple, cored (not peeled) and sliced into strips
200g peeled king prawns (defrosted if frozen)
3 tsp tamarind paste
1 red chilli, finely sliced
300–400g stir-fry vegetables – a mixture of whatever you fancy,
including beansprouts, julienned carrots, mushrooms, etc.
2 tbsp soy sauce
1 tbsp sesame oil
½ tsp Thai fish sauce

Cook the noodles according to the packet instructions and drain. Cut the florets off the broccoli and slice the stems. Heat 1 tbsp of oil in a large frying pan or wok, add the apple slices and stir-fry for three minutes. Transfer them to a plate. Add the prawns and two tsp of tamarind paste, and cook for 2–3 minutes. Remove and put aside with the apples. Add the remaining oil to the pan and stir-fry the chilli, vegetables and broccoli for four minutes. Add the prawns and apples to the pan and stir in the soy sauce, sesame oil, fish sauce and remaining tamarind. Cook for a couple of minutes and serve with the noodles.

Barley Chicken (serves 4)

4 chicken thighs, skinned and boned
3 tsp olive oil
1 onion, finely chopped
50g barley
50g puy lentils
2 tbsp chopped tarragon
750–1000ml vegetable or chicken stock

Chop the chicken meat into small cubes, trimming off the fat. Heat the oil in a pan over a medium heat. Add the onion and chicken pieces and fry until the onion is soft and the chicken is browned (about 5–7 minutes). Add the rest of the ingredients (750ml of stock to start with), lower the heat and simmer for 25–30 minutes until the liquid has gone. If the ingredients aren't quite cooked when the liquid has disappeared, add the rest of the stock and simmer for a little longer. Serve.

Carrot Veggie Burgers (makes 4–6)

splash of olive oil
1 onion, finely chopped
2 cloves of garlic, finely chopped
1 tsp ground coriander
2 tsp curry powder

400g can butterbeans, drained
1 handful of toasted walnuts or seeds
1 carrot, grated
fresh coriander, chopped
1 lime, zest and juice
seasoning
3–4 tbsp coconut milk
wholemeal plain flour

Heat the oil in a pan and lightly fry the onion until soft and translucent. Add the garlic, ground coriander and curry powder. Mix together and cook for a minute. Blend the spiced onions, beans and nuts/seeds in a food processer until well mixed, but not a smooth puree. Tip into a bowl. Mix in the carrot, fresh coriander, lime juice, grated zest, seasoning and coconut milk to bind. If the burgers are looking too wet, add more beans and some breadcrumbs. Shape into burgers. Dust your hands and burgers with the flour so things don't get too sticky. Sift flour over the burgers and place in the fridge for up to 2 hours before frying in a little oil or grilling.

Spicy Chops (serves 2)

2 decent-sized pork chops
1 orange, zest and juice
1 tbsp cumin seeds
1 tbsp paprika
pinch of cinnamon
pinch of chilli powder

Preheat your oven to 200°C/Gas 6. Pierce the chops with a fork and cover them with the orange zest and juice. Mix the spices together, along with a good pinch of pepper. Remove the chops from the juice, but reserve the liquid. Rub the spices well into the chops. Heat a frying pan with a little oil and cook gently on each side till just golden. Add the liquid to the pan and reduce a little. Put everything into a roasting tin and roast in the preheated oven for 10 minutes.

Salmon and Broccoli Noodles (serves 4)

2 tbsp lemon juice
1-inch cube of fresh ginger, peeled and chopped
4 cloves of garlic, chopped
1/3 tsp turmeric
pinch of chilli powder
4 salmon steaks
500g broccoli
250g rice noodles
chilli oil
seasoning

Mix the lemon juice, ginger, garlic, turmeric and chilli powder in a bowl and blend to a smooth paste. Place the salmon steaks in an ovenproof dish and smear the spice paste all over them. Set aside to marinate for 20 minutes. Boil a saucepan of water. Cut the florets from the broccoli into bite-sized pieces. Add to the boiling water. Cook for 2 minutes to soften. Turn off the heat and add the rice noodles, stirring briefly. Leave to stand for 1 minute. Strain the noodle mixture through a colander and transfer to a mixing bowl. Add a little chilli oil and seasoning, and toss. Set aside. Preheat the grill. Wipe the marinade off the salmon and place the fish on the grill pan, skin-side down. Grill on one side only for 3–5 minutes. Put the noodles and broccoli on serving plates and top with the salmon.

Rice Pasta with Smoked Salmon (serves 2)

3 tsp olive oil
1 clove of garlic, chopped
1 tsp capers, chopped
1 leek, finely sliced
1 large courgette, finely sliced
75g chopped mushrooms
2 tbsp white wine
2 tsp chopped tarragon
2 tbsp crème fraîche
150g smoked salmon, sliced
120 g rice (or vegetable) pasta

Heat the oil in a large pan and gently fry the garlic, capers, leek and courgette until soft (about 7–8 minutes). Add the mushrooms and cook for another 5 minutes, stirring regularly. Add the wine and simmer for a few minutes before adding the tarragon and crème fraîche. Add the salmon and lower the heat for 1 minute to warm through. As this is cooking, prepare the pasta. Drain well and add to the sauce. Serve immediately.

Tangy Swordfish (serves 4)

1 level tsp dried chilli flakes
4 tbsp olive oil
zest and juice of 1 lime, plus 1 whole lime, sliced, to serve
1 clove of garlic, crushed
4×175g swordfish steaks

Place the chilli flakes in a large shallow bowl. Add the olive oil, lime zest, juice and garlic and mix everything together. Add the swordfish steaks to the marinade and toss several times to coat completely. Leave to marinate for 30 minutes. Preheat a griddle pan until hot. Remove the swordfish from the marinade, season well, then cook the steaks for 2 minutes on each side. Top with slices of lime and continue to cook until the fish is opaque right through (1–2 minutes).

Thai Beef Salad (serves 2)

1 clove of garlic, chopped
1½ tsp brown sugar
1 tbsp lime juice
2 tbsp light soy sauce
½ cucumber
handful of beansprouts
1 red chilli, finely sliced
handful of mint leaves, chopped
1 little gem lettuce and other green leaves
2 sirloin or rump steaks

For the dressing: in a bowl, whisk the chopped garlic clove, brown sugar, lime juice and light soy sauce. Set aside. Cut the cucumber into sticks and put into a bowl. Add the beansprouts, the red chilli, mint leaves and the torn-up leaves of lettuce. Toss well and divide between two plates. Griddle, pan-fry or grill the seasoned steaks for 2–5 minutes each side. Place on a board and cut into slices, then divide between the plates and drizzle with the dressing.

Vegetable Stir-fry with Cashews (serves 4)

1 tsp groundnut oil

1 onion, peeled and sliced

1 clove of garlic, crushed

1 red pepper, deseeded and sliced

1 yellow pepper, deseeded and sliced

1 green pepper, deseeded and sliced

100g broccoli florets

175g baby sweetcorn

2 courgettes, sliced

50g water chestnuts, sliced

2 tbsp light soy sauce

1 tsp arrowroot mixed with 2 tbsp vegetable stock

2-inch piece of fresh ginger, grated

1 tbsp sweet chilli sauce

50g toasted cashews

Heat the oil in a wok and fry the onion and garlic for 3 minutes. Add the peppers and fry for 3 minutes more.

Add the broccoli florets, sweetcorn and courgettes and continue to fry for a further 5 minutes. Add the water chestnuts and toss to mix in. In a small bowl, mix together the soy sauce, arrowroot and light stock, ginger and sweet chilli sauce. Using a wooden spoon, make a space in the centre of the stir-fried vegetables so that the base of the wok is visible. Pour in the sauce and bring to the boil, stirring all the time until it starts to thicken. Toss the vegetables to coat thoroughly with the sauce. Transfer to a serving dish and sprinkle with the cashew nuts.

Salmon Fishcakes with Asparagus (serves 4)

500g potatoes, peeled and diced
3 salmon fillets, approx 350–400g
finely grated zest of ½ lemon
3 tbsp chopped fresh herbs – a mixture of dill leaves, parsley and tarragon is good
1 tbsp plain wholemeal flour
2 eggs, beaten
150g dried breadcrumbs
400g asparagus
splash of olive oil

Cook the potatoes in a pan of boiling water for 12–15 minutes. Drain, then mash and leave to cool. In the meantime, line a grill tray with foil and oil it lightly. Put the salmon on, skin-side down. Grill for around 8 minutes. Leave the salmon to cool, then flake, discarding the skin. Gently mix the flakes in a bowl with the potato, lemon zest, herbs and 1 tbsp flour. Mix in one of the beaten eggs. Divide the mixture into 6–8 evenly sized balls, and press into patties. Dust in a little more flour and chill for 30 minutes. Put the other egg and the breadcrumbs in separate flat dishes. Turn the fishcakes first in the egg, then the breadcrumbs to coat. Steam the asparagus for 5–8 minutes and at the same time fry the fishcakes for 3–4 minutes in a little oil until golden.

Portuguese-style Chicken (serves 4)

6–8 chicken pieces
1 tsp smoked paprika
1 tsp ground ginger
1 tsp dried oregano
1 tsp mild chilli powder
1 tsp salt
zest of 1 lime
pepper
2 heaped tbsp tomato purée
1 tbsp olive oil

Preheat the oven to 200°C/Gas 6. Trim most of the skin off the chicken pieces, leaving a top layer intact. Mix the smoked paprika, ginger, oregano, chilli powder, salt and lemon zest. Add a good grinding of pepper then mix in the tomato purée and olive oil to a thick paste. Throw in the chicken pieces and thoroughly coat, massaging the paste into every nook and cranny. Place in a non-stick roasting tin and cook in the oven for 40–45 minutes.

Coconut Vegetable Curry (serves 2–4)

1 cauliflower, cut into chunky pieces
2–3 handfuls of other seasonal veg, cut into chunks
splash of olive oil
2 cloves of garlic
1-inch cube of fresh ginger, peeled
½ fresh red or green chilli, roughly chopped
1 tsp turmeric
2 leeks, roughly chopped
1 heaped tsp peanut butter
1 lime, zest and juice
handful of fresh coriander
1 tbsp sesame oil
1 tbsp soy sauce
1 tin of coconut milk
250ml vegetable stock
handful of desiccated coconut, toasted

Preheat the oven to 200°C/Gas 6. Mix together the chopped vegetables and a splash of oil. Season. Roast in the preheated oven for 25 minutes. While that's cooking, put the garlic, ginger, chilli, turmeric, leek, peanut butter, lime juice and zest, coriander, sesame oil and soy sauce in a blender, to produce a paste. Add the coconut milk and stock to the paste. Blend to mix. Pour the sauce into the roasting tray over the roast veg. Cook for 5–10 minutes to warm the sauce. Serve with brown rice and a dusting of toasted coconut.

Seasonal Risotto (serves 4–6)

1 litre chicken or vegetable stock

1 tbsp olive oil

2 tbsp butter

1 onion, finely chopped

1 leek, finely chopped

1 celery stalk, finely chopped

1 clove of garlic, crushed

220g risotto rice (e.g. Arborio)

seasoning

150ml white wine

600g any seasonal mixed vegetables – e.g. courgettes, diced; French beans, chopped; asparagus spears, sliced; shelled fresh peas; broad beans; spinach leaves

1 tbsp freshly grated Parmesan cheese

1 tbsp chopped spring onions

Bring the stock to simmering point in a pan. Heat the olive oil and half the butter in a large, deep frying pan and add the onion, leek and celery. Cook gently for about 5 minutes, until soft, then stir in the garlic. Add the rice and turn up the heat a little. Season well and cook for a minute, stirring so the rice is coated with the fat. Add the white wine and cook until it has evaporated. Then start adding the hot stock a large spoonful at a time. Add the vegetables in order of cooking time (i.e. those that cook quickly, like spinach, should be added last). After the rice has been cooking for 15–18 minutes, check to see if it is cooked. When it is, take the pan off the heat and stir in the remaining butter and the Parmesan. Season to taste, then cover and allow to stand for 5–10 minutes. Sprinkle with the spring onions to serve.

Frittata Verdi (serves 2)

350g spinach, washed, with stalks removed
3 tbsp olive oil
1 onion, chopped
6 eggs
2 tbsp Parmesan or Gruyere cheese, grated
½ tsp nutmeg, grated
seasoning

Place the spinach into a pan of boiling water for 1 minute. Drain and cool in cold water. Squeeze dry, then chop finely. Heat 1 tbsp oil in a pan, add the onion and fry until soft. Mix with the spinach. Break the eggs into a bowl and add the cheese, spinach mixture and nutmeg. Season. Heat the rest of the oil in a large frying pan. Add the egg mixture and cook for about 5 minutes until starting to set. Place a large plate on top of the pan, turn the pan upside down so the frittata is on the plate, then tip back into the pan upside down and cook until the other side is just set. Cut into quarters and serve immediately.

9 Ice Exercise

Undoubtedly, one of the biggest factors contributing to weight problems is the amount of time we spend cooped up indoors. It's not just the warmth of the indoor environment that's hampering our health. It is what you do (or don't do) inside that is compounding the problem. The chances are that much of the time you are sitting down. Plenty of regular activity underpins the success of the Ice Diet; most of us do too little. We think we are more active than we are, but tot up the hours you spend on your backside and they probably exceed eight a day.

Environmental experts estimate that people living in developed countries now spend 90 per cent of their lives indoors. It's staggering, but in reality the figure is often closer to nudging 98 per cent, for how many people do you know who spend two and a half hours outside every day? Unless you have a job that demands you are on your feet or outdoors, the likelihood is that you sit down at work, in the car and in front of the TV in the evening, moving only to shift from one indoor seat to another. Think about it. We work indoors, we drive everywhere. We increasingly shop either online or in huge indoor shopping malls. With around 8 million people paying to be a member of a private gym or health club, many of us even prefer to exercise with a roof over our heads than to head out for a walk, a cycle or a run.

Being seated burns a bare minimum of calories – even eating an apple or fidgeting uses more energy than parking your bottom on a chair – and it is almost inevitable that long-term sitters find they get fatter. Emerging research suggests that there are also more sinister happenings when we sit down for too long. Studies on rats have shown that substances that play a crucial role in metabolizing fat and sugar in the body are only produced when muscles are being used, even if that's just standing up.

Prolonged sitting has been linked to a sharp reduction in the activity of an important enzyme called lipoprotein lipase, which breaks down blood fats and makes them available as a fuel to the muscles. This reduction in enzyme activity leads to raised levels of triglycerides and fats in the blood, increasing the risk of heart disease. Add to that the fact that extended sitting has been shown to cause sharp spikes in blood sugar levels after meals, creating the perfect physiological setting for Type 2 diabetes and there is a huge case for getting up and getting outside.

There are more subtle ways in which our attempts to lose weight are thwarted by being inside so much. One example is the lack of stairs we are exposed to in new buildings, something that concerns physical activity researchers tremendously. Dr Oliver Webb, a sports scientist at Loughborough University, conducted a large study looking at the availability of stairs in newly built shopping malls, airports and other public places around the UK.[1] There were pitifully few. Instead he found that architects are designing these centres with escalators and lifts to comply with access requirements, making stairs a secondary consideration. Even when there are stairs, they are often hidden from view. And because they are not visible, people opt for the lift instead.

Outdoors, we are not only exposed to fluctuations in temperature, but to unpredictable terrain and physical challenges. We climb and descend steps and kerbs without realizing it. We swerve to manoeuvre around other shoppers as we power walk down the high street to dodge the rain. We put on a spurt to reach a crossing in time to make it before the lights change. In short, the outdoors is a ready-made and far more effective gym and weight-loss mechanism than any indoor fitness emporium we pay to belong to.

How Hot is Your Gym?

Around 8 million people are now members of private gyms and health clubs in the UK. It's commendable that so many are taking a step towards greater levels of activity. But is indoors really the best place to exercise? One of my main gripes about gyms (and the number-one complaint by regular users in many surveys) is that they are invariably too hot. Summer months aside – when the air conditioning is blasted out – before you even begin to think about working out at my local gym between September and April, you are liable to break into a sweat. It is so hot you feel as if you barely need a warm-up to prepare yourself for more intense effort: you would heat up even in a crop-top. Changing rooms are stuffy and workout areas are stifling, with barely an open window to be seen.

Some are hotter than others. In my experience, council-owned gyms are less heated than private health clubs, presumably because it costs so much to maintain such a cocoon of warmth in which to exercise. There are no official limits to how hot a gym can be, but the International Fitness Association suggests that areas near pools be kept between 21 and 26 °C, and to maintain aerobics, cardio, weight-training and Pilates rooms at approximately 18 to 20 °C. Humidity levels for all areas should be around 40 to 60 per cent. In reality, though, temperatures are often hotter than this. It makes for an uncomfortable environment in which to exercise and also minimizes the body's ability to activate good brown fat.

Take the Heat Out of Your Workout

The fitness industry is largely built on the concept that getting hot and sweating as a consequence is good for us. Gyms like us to believe that heat and perspiration gets you fitter. Sweat has become a byword for clean living and sound health. It's an ideal that makes us want to buy clothes from Sweaty Betty or running shoes from the Sweat Shop. And it's why we want to finish a run dripping like Sylvester Stallone's Rocky or Matthew McConaughy in one of his perspiration-soaked roles.

Heated exercise pods are all the rage in the US, the idea

being that your body gets more benefit from stretching and working against resistance when it's stifling. And we see an endless stream of heated workouts – from hot Pilates to hot spinning – on the timetables of gyms. Classes are held in rooms heated to 27–28 °C. And, of course, there's hot yoga, which is sold on the fact that the heat – up to an oppressive 40 °C – offers untold benefits, including the fact that the temperature of the room makes you work harder and sweat away extra calories.

Whether or not heat does enhance workouts is highly questionable. My background in sports science tells me that it is not a sensible move to push yourself in hot temperatures as it raises heart rate and blood pressure, which can be a risky combination, and this is confirmed by experts I have consulted. More than that, there are doubts about whether it actually gets you any fitter. In a study at the University of Wisconsin,[2] exercise physiologists conducted regular tests to compare the workout intensity of regular yoga in a non-heated room with the hot yoga approach.

Results revealed startling similarities of effort. In hot yoga, the exercise intensity of those taking part was an average 57 per cent of maximal heart rate compared to 56 per cent in basic yoga, levels that fitness industry guidelines would classify as 'light' exercise, barely more physically demanding than a gentle walk. Cedric Bryant, Chief Scientific Officer for the non-profit-making US consumer watchdog, the American Council on Exercise (ACE), said the benefits of the heat are largely perceptual. 'People think the degree of sweat is the quality of the workout, but that's not the reality,' Dr Bryant says. 'Heat doesn't correlate to burning more calories.'

Hot yoga is sold on the fact that the heat offers untold benefits, including eliminating the need for an extended warm-up so that more time can be devoted to the classic series of twenty-six postures and two breathing exercises. There is an element of truth in the notion that the heat may mean the muscles, tendons and ligaments are more flexible in much the same way as they are after a thorough warm-up. However, overall suppleness is dependent on connective tissue and heat doesn't play an important role in improving it. Heat has no hidden advantage when it comes to improving balance, strength, endurance or all-round fitness. Heat, in itself, is not going to fast-track you into your bikini.

If heat doesn't help us burn calories when we exercise, what does it do? The truth is that while sweat is important, its benefits are hugely overplayed. It's crucial as the body's heat-control mechanism, as a vital means of keeping the body cool, but not as a means of flushing away unwanted chemicals or anything else. We certainly don't need to sweat more by getting extra hot when we exercise; we can afford to sweat less. The idea that dripping sweat is somehow healthy is a fallacy. It's the evaporation of sweat from the body that cools you; working out in a hot environment just makes it more difficult for that evaporation to occur. Any extra weight lost will be marginal and comprise fluid losses that will be replaced as soon as you drink to rehydrate.

Getting outside as often as you can is key to the success

of the Ice Diet and long-term healthy living. Still need convincing? The following should provide the evidence to sway you.

Six Reasons to Exercise Outdoors

1. A review of studies at the University of Exeter[3] in which volunteers were asked to do two walks of about the same time or distance either inside on a treadmill or outdoors revealed an almost unanimous preference for the outdoor version. Subsequent psychological tests showed the hikers scored significantly higher on measures of enthusiasm, revitalization and self-esteem, whereas those stuck indoors had higher feelings of tension, depression and fatigue.

2. Psychologists at the University of Essex[4] reported that 'green exercise' in which people are exposed to natural environments leads to lower rates of perceived exertion – in other words, they feel like they aren't working as hard as in other surroundings.

3. A report commissioned by the Countryside Recreation Network found that self-esteem was significantly boosted and more weight lost in nine out of ten people who switched from exercising indoors to out.[5] And the Mental Health Foundation says outdoor activity provides a sense of accomplishment people don't report after working out at an indoor gym.

4. Vitamin-D levels are worryingly low in people who don't get outside much. Food supplies of this important

nutrient are scarce; by far the most efficient source is the sun as it is synthesized when chemicals in the skin react to ultraviolet rays. Dr Graeme Close, a researcher in sports nutrition and exercise metabolism at Liverpool John Moores University, has found that our indoor workout habits compound the lack of vitamin D available to our bodies. Gwyneth Paltrow, known for her dedication to fitness almost as much as for her acting, is among those to have been diagnosed as vitamin-D deficient a few years ago.

5. Reduce the amount of clothing you wear to exercise outdoors and you not only implement an important cooling strategy, but get an added bonus. Dr Close says that people who wear tight-fitting base layers and compression-type clothing are also limiting their skin's exposure to daylight, reducing the amount of vitamin D produced in the body. Using even conservative guidelines, up to 70 per cent of the recreational and serious athletes tested by Dr Close are found to have worryingly low vitamin-D levels partly because of this.

6. Scientists have proven that we have an innate attraction to Nature called biophilia – and that reverting back to our ancestors' habits of being outside more often can boost mental and physical health. Work from Japan and the Netherlands has shown that just having access to an open space means people live longer and enjoy better health. In one experiment it was shown how patients recovering from identical operations were more likely to get better quickly, need fewer painkillers and have fewer

side effects if they could only see the outdoors from their bedside.

Top Ice Diet Workouts

Walking

Long-derided as the poor relation to running, walking is coming into its own as an essential element of the A-lister's exercise regimen. Charlize Theron, Uma Thurman and Jessica Biel are among those who have recently credited walking with helping them to stay in shape. It's hard to find an activity with a greater celebrity following or, indeed, the barrage of research that walking has to support it. It's been shown to reduce cancer death risk by up to 34 per cent and cut your risk of Type 2 diabetes in half.

Of course, there is nothing better than a walk on a cold winter's day to enhance your cool lifestyle. But walking in any weather brings benefits and not just to your waistline. Regular brisk walking can lower your risk of high blood pressure, high cholesterol and diabetes as much as running can, according to some researchers. Adding 2,000 moderately paced walking steps (or 20 minutes) a day to regular activity could help people to cut their risk of heart attacks and strokes by 8 per cent; doing 4,000 more steps (40 minutes of added walking), matches the gains obtained from taking cholesterol-lowering drugs.

The speed you walk at also determines how much energy you will burn – the faster you move, the greater the calorie-gobbling will be. In half an hour, a 9½-stone person will use up 75 calories on a 2mph stroll, 99 calories if the pace is increased to 3mph and 150 calories on a brisk 4mph stride-out. It doesn't need to be flat out all the way – the interval-style walks prescribed in the Ice Diet 6-Week Plan in which you incorporate fast and slow bursts of effort are extremely effective at improving cardiovascular fitness and boosting your metabolism very quickly.

Style is important if you are going to make walking the mainstay of your fitness routine. Practice by walking at a comfortable pace and focusing on your posture by lifting up through the centre of your body, relaxing your shoulders down and swinging your arms in rhythm with your stride. Your arm swing should be from the shoulder (rather than the elbow) and your arms should not cross the centre line of the body. The length of each stride should be comfortable and, on planting your heel, the toes should be raised towards the shins. Next, the foot rolls from heel to toe and then pushes off. In recent years, runners have been encouraged to alter their technique by landing on the forefoot with each stride to avoid injuries. A study in the *Journal of Experimental Biology*[6] looked at the ergonomics of walking and found walking heel to toe is more efficient for humans. Of twenty-seven volunteers asked to walk on a treadmill, those aiming to land on the balls of their feet used 50 per cent more effort than heel-to-toe walkers. Those on tiptoe not only looked ridiculous but expended 83 per cent more effort than the heel-to-toe rollers despite burning no more calories.

For faster-paced walking and HIIT-style spurts (see below), you'll need to tweak your technique. Concentrate on increasing stride frequency, not stride length, and pumping your arms; a high lift behind the elbows will particularly assist this. On contact, exaggerate the lift of the toes and move smoothly from the heel to the ball of the foot in a continuous rolling motion, adding a strong push off your big toe. To help increase speed, narrow your stride width a little, like walking on a tightrope rather than train lines. Lean forwards from your ankles as this will give you a feeling of being able to push harder against the ground. It will also help you to avoid the over-striding that can slow you down.

Outdoor HIIT

High Intensity Interval Training, or HIIT, has become accepted as one of the most effective ways to boost your fitness and, some studies have shown,[7] can enhance the production of calorie-burning good fat. It was the subject of *Fast Exercise*, a book I wrote with Dr Michael Mosley, which shot to the top of the bestseller list on both sides of the Atlantic.[8] The appeal is simple: it's tough but quick and over before you know it, sometimes even before you have time to break into a sweat. An editor of a glossy magazine claims she completes her HIIT session in her work clothes and doesn't even have to shower or change when it's done.

In my experience, it demands more than that and I am invariably floored when it's over. But there's little doubt it's a great addition to the Ice Diet plan. First murmurings of its benefits came seven years ago when studies at McMaster University in Ontario showed that 30-second bike sprints for a total of 3 minutes led to the same muscle-cell adaptations as two hours of long, steady bike riding.[9] Since then, dozens of research papers have shown that it's not the duration of a workout that matters, but the gut-busting effort you are prepared to make while doing it.

For top athletes, HIIT-style training has been part and parcel of weekly preparation for many decades. Indeed, there is unlikely to be anyone who reaches the top in sport without making this sort of training part of their workload. Many of the daily activities included in the 6-Week Ice Diet Plan are based on HIIT principles. But the variety of what you can include knows no bounds. Once you have reached a certain level of fitness, you too can push on to the next level. You will notice that your muscles become more defined, your body fat drops and your aerobic endurance also improves. What I like most about it is the dramatic effect it can have on your performance in sports and other activities. In my case, I can clearly see how just a few weeks of HIIT boosts not only my fat-burning, but my speed at running – my own favourite activity.

There is no hard and fast rule as to how long a HIIT session should last, other than it should be at least 1 minute, but no longer than 10 minutes. Exercise scientists at Abertay University in Dundee have shown that, in addition to daily activities like walking, just 60 seconds of effort – sprint all-out for 6 seconds on a bike then rest for one minute, repeating the cycle ten times, three times a week – is all a middle-aged person needs to enhance their health status.[10] Others have demonstrated how the 3-minute approach – a 20-second flat-out sprint followed by a 2-minute recovery, repeated three times – is a short but effective workout.

Fashionable New Yorkers are currently into the 7-Minute Workout, a bodyweight circuit with twelve exercises including the plank, lunges and push-ups, that was shown in a study published in the journal of the American College of Sports Medicine to produce results comparable to a run-and-weights session combined.[11] Or you could try the single 4-minute fast run shown in Norwegian trials to boost endurance and general fitness. When performed three times a week, the 4-minute pelter was enough to boost the health and fitness of middle-aged men significantly. At the end of a ten-week trial, they had lost a few pounds, lowered their blood pressure and improved their blood sugar control.[12]

What I love most about HIIT is that it can be performed outdoors and adapted to weather conditions and your environment. I use natural markers to 'plot' my session – trees, benches and even lamp posts – varying the terrain on which I run, walk or cycle (my preferred modes of activity). Dirt trails, grass, pavements, pine needles, uphills and downhills all place different demands on the body and muscles, requiring you to change rhythm and speed, and, above all, keep things interesting.

Below is a 2-week 'Ice Blast' programme that is great for maximizing fat burning in conjunction with the Ice Diet. It is not for the faint-hearted or those who are new to exercise, but is a great regimen for those of you with a decent fitness base who want a hard-hitting kick-start.

Ice Blast HIIT Programme

The Exercises

Burpees

Start in a crouched position with knees tucked in and hands on the floor. Kick your legs powerfully behind you so that they are straight, then jump them back between your arms to the start position in a quick movement. Immediately leap up into the air, swinging your arms directly above your head to give you height. Return to the crouched starting position and repeat.

Jumping Jacks

Stand with your hands by your sides. In one movement, jump up, spreading your legs apart as you raise your arms over your head. You should land with your arms over your head and your feet more than hip-width apart. Jump up again and, in one movement, bring your legs together and your arms back to your sides. You have just done one jumping jack. Keep going for 30 seconds.

Lateral Jumps

Place a marker on the floor – I use a bar, but you can use anything from a cone to a handbag. Stand beside the marker, side on and about 40–50cm away from it. With your feet hip-width apart, bend your knees to 90 degrees and pull your shoulders back slightly. Place your arms in front of you. Then explode up and over the marker, throwing your arms behind you to propel you. As you jump into the air, keep your feet level with each other and parallel with the floor. Try to land softly and quietly on the mid-foot, rolling into the heels. Push your hips back and down to absorb the impact of landing. Do not lock out your knees. Repeat, jumping back in the opposite direction.

Squat Thrusts

Start as you would for a push-up with legs outstretched behind you, arms wider than shoulder-width and straight, hands on the floor directly beneath your shoulders and your weight on the balls of your feet or your toes. Quickly jump both legs forward, bending your knees so that your knees are tucked between your arms and you land on the mid-feet. Jump both legs back to the starting position and repeat.

High-knee Running

Stand tall and begin jogging either on the spot or forward. Without leaning back, drive through the balls of your feet and try to bring your knees close to chest level. Keep your hands relaxed, elbows bent and shoulders down, and swing your arms back and forth to help you keep going. Again, 30 seconds of this is hard work. Start slow.

Knee-tuck Crossovers

Start as you would for a push-up with legs outstretched behind you, arms wider than shoulder-width and straight, hands on the floor directly beneath your shoulders and weight on the balls of your feet or your toes. Lift your left foot off the floor and bend at the knee, bringing it underneath the body to reach towards your right arm. Don't twist your back. Slowly return to the start position and repeat on the other side.

Jump Squats

Start with feet shoulder-width apart, knees bent and bottom sticking out in a squat position. Allow your arms to hang by your sides and keep your back straight. Simultaneously push through your heels and swing up your arms to leap upward as high as you can. Land softly on the balls of your feet, rolling through to your heels. Repeat.

Step Up and Press

For this you will need a dumb-bell or a bottle of water and a sturdy bench or chair. Decide which leg you are going to step up with first and hold the weight in the opposite hand. Place one foot on the 'step', making sure your whole foot is in contact with the surface. Push your body weight up, driving your weight through your heel and breathing out as you do this. At the same time, push or press the weight up towards the ceiling until your arm is straight. Step back and down, one leg at a time, until you are standing with both feet flat on the floor again. Repeat on the same side for half the specified repetitions and then switch legs and arms.

The Workouts

Week 1

Day 1: 20-minute run or cycle incorporating 5 × 20-second sprints.

Day 2: REST.

Day 3: 30 seconds each of burpees, jumping jacks, squat thrusts, high-knee running, jump squats, step up and press, lateral jumps and knee-tuck crossovers with 10 seconds rest between each. Repeat.

Day 4: Warm up, then perform 4×60-second sprints on the bike or running with a 90-second breather. Cool down for 3–4 minutes.

Day 5: Warm up, 5 × 30-second sprints uphill on bike or running. Cool down.

Day 6: 10× each of burpees, jumping jacks, lateral jumps and step up and presses with a 10-second breather between each. Then take a 20-second breather and repeat each

9 times, then a 20-second breather and perform each 8 times, etc., until you perform just one repetition of each.
Day 7: Warm up. Sprint for 30 seconds, rest for 15 seconds. Repeat 8 times. Cool down.

Week 2

Day 1: 20-minute run or cycle with 6×20-second sprints.
Day 2: REST.
Day 3: 30 seconds of burpees, jumping jacks, squat thrusts, high-knee running, jump squats, step up and presses, lateral jumps and knee-tuck crossovers with 10 seconds rest between each. Repeat.
Day 4: 10 minutes easy running, 3 minutes hard, 5 minutes easy.
Day 5: 10× each of burpees, jumping jacks, lateral jumps and step up and presses with a 10-second breather between each. Then take a 20-second breather and repeat each 9 times, then a 20-second breather and each 8 times, etc., until you perform just one repetition of each.
Day 6: Warm up, run or cycle 60 seconds hard, 90 seconds easy. Repeat 6 times. Cool down.
Day 7: 30 seconds of burpees, jumping jacks, squat thrusts, high-knee running, jump squats, step up and presses, lateral jumps and knee-tuck crossovers with 10 seconds rest between each. Repeat.

What Happens When You Hit the Dreaded Fitness Plateau?

Whichever approach you choose, there will come a time when your body adapts to the effort you are putting into it and will not respond as well as it did a few weeks previously. In other words, you hit the dreaded fitness plateau. It's at this point that you need to make tweaks to your regime, to raise your workouts to the next level so that your body begins to respond again. This does not necessarily mean you have to increase the duration of your exercise dramatically – progression can be achieved by increasing the intensity or speed of your 'efforts', by attempting to complete more moves in an allotted time or by shortening recovery time so that you can attempt a greater number of fast 'bursts'.

Evolutionary Fitness

A few years ago the concept of crawling through leaves and squatting like a gorilla might have seemed an inconceivable alternative to a step aerobics class. But a general swell of anti-gym sentiment among those, like me, who are disillusioned with its overheated and sterile environment has already seen a burgeoning trend for a more organic approach to working out. And 'evolutionary exercise' is among the most enjoyable and effective forms of exercise to emerge from this branch of fitness.

In a nutshell, the evolutionary approach to workouts aims to reintroduce the natural movement patterns – crawling, jumping, lifting and climbing – that kept our ancestors strong and agile before the advent of plush gyms and yoga studios. The idea is simple: turn nature into your fitness emporium by using stones as dumb-bells, branches as pull-up bars and logs as steppers.

Enthusiasts believe that many of the aches and ailments that have become part and parcel of modern living – back pain, bad posture and knee pain – are the result of constrained and repetitive movement. At gyms, we exercise mindlessly and across limited planes, rarely challenging our bodies in new ways. We swing Kettlebells, but in the same ways, week in, week out. We run on treadmills that offer nothing in the way of the variety that you get outside.

Such habitual motion puts strain on the same muscles and joints, causing problems such as overuse injuries, but it also fails to stimulate the mind. We have a primal need to challenge ourselves physically. Below are some of my favourite 'evolutionary' moves, but by all means add your own. You don't need to live in the 'wilds' to take it up. I first tried it in a central London park with an instructor who opened my eyes to a whole new world of exercise. Part of the fun is discovering how your body can use and adapt to the environment to get stronger and fitter.

Deep Squat

Stretches and works the muscles in the buttocks and legs. Stand with feet wider than hip-width apart and back straight. Bend your knees to drop down into as deep a squat as possible with your buttocks aiming for the ground. The position should feel relaxed and you should keep your heels on the ground. Allow your arms to hang in front of the body and keep your head in line with the spine. If you find this too difficult at first, try holding on to a bench or tree for support. Hold the position for 15–60 seconds.

Hang and Swing

Targets rarely used muscles in the upper back and shoulders as well as the abdominals and arms. Find a horizontal branch within easy reach. From a standing position, jump up and grab the branch and hang from it for 15–30 seconds. As you get fitter, progress to swinging forward and backwards or from side to side. Try to move your hands along the branch travelling left to right using your back, hips and knees to gain momentum.

Throw and Sprint

Develops arm and leg strength as well as speed and power. Find something to throw – a stick, a small rock – and throw it as far as you can ahead of you, rocking your body weight and using plenty of arm and upper-body rotation to generate power. When it lands, sprint to fetch it. Repeat 6–10 times, alternating the throwing arm.

Log Haul

This can be performed with a log or rock that is heavy enough to require effort but not so heavy that it is a strain to lift. Squat down from the knees (keeping back straight) to pick up the item and lift it, preferably to shoulder level. If it's too heavy, carry it with straight arms, keeping good spinal alignment. Carry it a distance of 10–20 metres, aiming to move as quickly as possible. Repeat 5–8 times.

Bear Crawl

Provides an entire body workout and is great to warm up for a circuit. Start on all fours and begin moving along the ground as quickly as you can. Add variations – move the arm and leg from the same side of the body at the same time (ipsilateral movement), the opposite arm and foot (contralateral) or move sideways. Keep the hips straight and low at first (as if stalking something in a bush) and then change to a high-level crawl. Continue for 2–3 minutes.

Swimming

If many gyms are hot, then indoor pools are scorching. Tropically warm waters seem to be a more common feature of private health clubs, but no pool is immune. It's far from unusual to dip a toe in waters of 29 °C (widely considered the recommended upper limit for recreational swimmers) up to 35 °C or higher in a hotel or health club pool, in excess of the 25–28 °C set by FINA, the international governing body of swimming, and by the Red Cross and British Swimming, as the perfect temperature for competitive and fitness swimming.

Nobody would dispute that diving into a pleasantly heated swimming pool is a more pleasurable experience than the 'catch-your-breath' shock of a cold dip. Once you start to swim, though, the warmth impedes your progress in a number of ways. When I was at university I shared a house with a group of friends, one of whom was an elite swimmer who competed at international level and trained with Olympic gold medallists. How they hated warm water. It was a persistent topic of conversation, a regular moan when the water of the pool where they trained was raised even by tiny increments in temperature.

Why is this? Hotter water makes swimming harder work. It increases all of the physiological parameters of performance. A swimmer going flat out in the pool has to work harder in warmer water to maintain a high level of effort.[13] Even for pool plodders like myself, there are downsides to too-warm pools. As water temperature rises, so does heart rate, largely because the effort required by the body to dissipate heat generated in a swim is raised.

Serious swimmers see overly warm pools as potentially risky in a number of ways: they can raise the likelihood of dehydration, muscle cramps and overheating of the body. Water chemistry is another factor that comes into play: treating warm water with chemicals is fraught with difficulty. The warmer the pool water, the less effective the chlorine-based disinfectants are.

Bacteria, algae and other organisms thrive in warm, wet conditions, one of the reasons why hot tubs are the number-one spot in a gym for catching an infection. British Swimming says the proliferation of bacteria as micro-organisms multiply faster in warm water – up to twice as fast for a rise of 10 °C – which means that filters in warmer pools are increasingly likely to be colonized.[14]

Obviously, babies (who have difficulty regulating body temperature) and people with disabilities or those having pool-based therapies need warmer temperatures than the rest of us. But if you are swimming for leisure and fitness, my advice is to choose a pool that is cool. It may be that you head outdoors to the increasing number of lidos that are being refurbished around the country. I am a regular user of my nearest and can vouch for them not just because they provide a far more appropriate temperature in which to get the most out of your swimming, but as a thoroughly more pleasant experience all round.

An alternative for the stronger and more adventurous is open-water swimming. For years associated with the batty bunch who plunge into the Serpentine on New Year's Day, this is an activity that has come into its own with a colossal and ever-growing number of participants. It's important to point out that there is a risk to swimming in too-cold waters for some people. If you have existing heart problems or any long-term medical issues, then the relative warmth of a lido is probably best for you. Diving into cold-water immersion triggers a shock response that can cause hyperventilation and a racing heart. It's no coincidence that many of the deaths in triathlons occur during the open-swim phase of the event and predominantly among relative newcomers to the sport. These deaths can often be loosely linked to previously undetected heart problems, the most plausible theory being that the open-water swim triggers a particular type of cardiac arrhythmia caused by a genetic condition called 'long QT syndrome'. In short, it's worth a medical overhaul if you do want to take it up.

For the nervous, there is no better place to start than the Outdoor Swimming Society (outdoorswimmingsociety.com), an organization that provides reams of advice and practical tips for those looking to dip their toe into open waters for the first time, and to do it safely. They hold training and competitive group swims in rivers, lakes and seas around the UK. The society's manifesto states that it's time swimmers had more fun and that swimmers 'have too long been held in chlorinated captivity – everyone with a set of bathers should be set free to immerse themselves in nature'. I couldn't agree more. Looking at the roof of a swimming pool or a clear blue sky as you do your lengths? In my book, there is no comparison.

10 Troubleshooting

Will I crave comfort foods?

A lot of people claim to crave stodgy foods like steamed puddings, mashed potatoes and cheese, and other high-calorie, high-carb dishes that make them feel warm and cosy when it's cold outside. But while comfort eaters claim their instincts are a throwback to the days when people needed extra layers of body fat to survive the winter, as you have read, food was scarce in the cold months for our ancestors. They certainly didn't have bowls of rice pudding on standby.

Instead, comfort eating comes down to modern physiology and the way our bodies respond to colder weather. If you are living a warm lifestyle, then any drop in temperature will come as a shock to your body, triggering the same self-preservation response that sends the body a message to heat up fast. You might turn up the heating or indulge in the sugars and starches that provide the instant 'heat' boost your body is longing for. Gradually acclimatize to colder temperatures in the way the Ice Diet recommends and those cravings will disappear.

Why am I finding it hard to adapt to cooling?

Rule number one is to take things slowly so that you experience minimal discomfort. Cold air is easier to tolerate than cold water, so opening windows, getting outside on a cold day or wearing fewer clothes on a mild morning are all great starting points. When it comes to water, I am not one to advocate cold showers. However, I found that splashing my face with cold water in the morning was a really good way to begin the acclimatization process. It also woke me up and was incredibly refreshing. From there, add splashes of cooler water to your back and then the front of your torso in the shower. Small steps will help you much more effectively than giant strides.

How do I know if I am too cold too soon?

There's a short answer to this: you will start to shiver. Your body's in-built temperature regulator is the best gauge you have to monitoring your own cooling strategies. If you are outside in the cool air and you start to shiver, add a layer.

I'm finding it hard to reduce my 'eating window'.

Again, take your time. There is no race to achieve two meals a day in eight hours. In fact, as outlined earlier, it may be that a more lenient approach suits your lifestyle and supports your activity levels better. After months of experimenting, I know that around 15:9 is best for me. But there is no hard and fast rule here. Use the guidelines to find what best suits your own body.

Where can I try cryotherapy?

As you've read, cryotherapy units are hugely popular with elite sports teams and football clubs. West Ham United

Sports Science Department says: 'We have found that the players report feeling fresher after entering the chamber, and are more than happy to do so. Cryotherapy has become an important part of our recovery process.' And the Head of Physical Performance at Welsh Rugby Union is equally glowing in his recommendation: 'It helps the players recover quicker from very intensive training sessions while assisting them complete a higher volume block of training. The enhanced recovery benefits definitely contribute to being able to enhance levels of fitness.'

There are numerous companies that offer cryotherapy to the general public or who provide access via mobile cryotherapy pods, including the following: Ice Health (icehealth.co.uk); Mobile Cryotherapy (boconline.co.uk); spas such as the exclusive Penny Hill Park in Surrey, where the England rugby team train, who offer a user-friendly variation called 'ice caves' and also advocate boosting circulation by rubbing the body with fresh, crushed ice from ice fountains (pennyhillpark.co.uk).

Where can I get hold of an ice vest?

Lots of sports companies now make ice-cooling vests. Among the best I've come across are the Australian-designed Arctic Heat Cooling Vest (uksportsproducts.com), and the Koolmax jacket and accessories (polarproducts. com).

References

1 Ice Power

1. Department of Energy and Climate Change, 'UK Housing Energy Fact File, 2014', January 2014.
2. HomeServe survey, uswitch.com, January 2014.
3. npower 'Big Switch On' survey, 2013.
4. J. J. Massen, K. Dusch, O. T. Eldakar, A. C. Gallup, 'A thermal window for yawning in humans: Yawning as a brain cooling mechanism', *Physiology & Behaviour*, vol. 130 (May 2014), pp. 145–8.
5. Raymond J. Cronise, David A. Sinclair, Andrew A. Bremer, 'The "Metabolic Winter" hypothesis: A cause of the current epidemics of obesity and cardiometabolic disease', *Metabolic Syndrome and Related Disorders*, vol. 12, issue 7 (2014).
6. F. Johnson, A. Mavrogianni, M. Ucci, A. Vidal-Puig, J. Wardle, 'Could increased time spent in a thermal comfort zone contribute to population increases in obesity?' *Obesity Reviews*, vol. 12, issue 7 (July 2011).
7. P. Lee, J. D. Linderman, S. Smith, R. J. Brychta, J. Wang, C. Idelson, R. M. Perron, C. D. Werner, G. Q. Phan, U. S. Kammula, E. Kebebew, K. Pacak, K. Y. Chen, F. S. Celi, 'Irsin and FGF21 are cold-induced endocrine activators of brown fat functions in humans', *Cell Metabolism*, vol. 19, issue 2 (2014), pp. 302–309.

8. Wouter van Marken Lichtenbelt, Boris Kingma, Anouk van der Lans, Lisje Schellen, 'Cold exposure – an approach to increasing expenditure in humans', *Trends in Endocrinology & Metabolism*, vol. 25, issue 4 (2014).

9. T. Yoneshiro, S. Aita, M. Matsushita, T. Kayahara, T. Kameya, Y. Kawai, T. Iwanaga, M. Saito, 'Recruited brown adipose tissue as an antiobesity agent in humans', *Journal of Clinical Investigation*, vol. 123, issue 8 (August 2013).

10. A. van der Lans, J. Hoeks, B. Brans, G. Vijgen, M. G. W. Visser, M. J. Vosselman, J. Hansen, J. A. Jörgensen, J. Wu, F. M. Mottaghy, P. Schrauwen, W. D. van Marken Lichtenbelt, 'Cold aclimation recruits human brown fat and increases non-shivering thermogenesis', *Journal of Clinical Investigation*, vol. 123, issue 8 (2013).

11. P. Lee, S. Smith, J. Linderman, A. B. Courville, R. J. Brychta, W. Dieckmann, C. D. Werner, K. Y. Chen, F. S. Celi, 'Temperature-acclimated brown adipose tissue modulates insulin sensitivity in humans', *Diabetes* (22 June, 2014).

12. 'The Rise of Home Fever', Allergy UK (2011).

13. S. Shefi, P. E. Tarapore, T. J. Walsh, M. Croughan, P. J. Turek, 'Wet heat exposure: a potentially reversible cause of low semen quality in infertile men', *Int. Braz. J. Urol.*, vol. 33, issue 1 (Jan/Feb. 2007).

14. N. A. Shevchuk, 'Adapted cold shower as a potential treatment for depression', *Med. Hypothesis*, vol. 70, issue 5 (November 2008).

15. R. Sellaro, B. Hommel, M. Manaï, L. S. Colzato, 'Preferred, but not objective temperature predicts working memory depletion', *Psychological Research* (2014) (epub).

16. Thermogenex, hypothermics.com.

17. Han Kim, Clark Richardson, Jeanette Roberts, Lisa Gren, Joseph L. Lyon, 'Cold Hands, Warm Heart', *The Lancet*, volume 351, issue 9114 (May 1988).

18. P. Tikuisis, I. Jacobs, D. Moroz, A. L. Vallerand, L. Martineau, 'Comparison of thermoregulatory responses between men and women immersed in cold water', *Journal of Applied Physiology*, volume 89, issue 4 (October 2000).

2 Good Fat, Bad Fat

1. A. M. Cypess, S. Lehman, G. Williams, I. Tal, D. Rodman, A. B. Goldfine, F. C. Kuo, E. L. Palmer, Y. Tseng, A. Doria, G. M. Kolodny, C. R. Kahn, 'Identification and importance of brown adipose tissue in adult humans', *New England Journal of Medicine*, vol. 360, issue 15 (2009).

2. Kirsi A. Virtanen, Martin E. Lidell, Janne Orava, Mikael Heglind, Rickard Westergren, Tarja Niemi, Markku Taittonen, Jukka Laine, Nina-Johanna Savisto, Sven Enerbäck, Pirjo Nuutila, 'Functional brown adipose tissue in healthy adults', *New England Journal of Medicine*, vol. 360, issue 15 (2009).

3. W. D. van Marken Lichtenbelt, Joost W. Vanhommerig, Nanda M. Smulders, Jamie M. A. F. L. Drossaerts, Gerrit J. Kemerink, Nicole D. Bouvy, Patrick Schrauwen, G. J. Jaap Teule, 'Cold-activated brown adipose tissue in healthy men', *New England Journal of Medicine*, vol. 360, issue 15 (2009).

4. E. Ravussin, L. P. Kozak, 'Have we entered the brown adipose tissue renaissance?', *Obesity Review*, vol. 10, issue 3 (May 2009).

5. H. Sacks, M. E. Symonds, 'Anatomical locations of human brown adipose tissue; functional relevance and implications in obesity and type 2 diabetes', *Diabetes*, vol. 62, issue 6 (June 2013).

6. P. Lee, S. Smith, J. Linderman, A. B. Courville, R. J. Brychta, W. Dieckmann, C. D. Werner, K. Y. Chen, F. S. Celi, 'Temperature-acclimated brown adipose tissue modulates insulin sensitivity in humans', *Diabetes* (22 June, 2014) (epub).

7. Narendra L. Reddy, Terence A. Jones, Sarah C. Wayte, Oludolapo Adesanya, Sailesh Sankar, Yen C. Yeo, Gyanendra Tripathi, Philip G. McTernan, Harpal S. Randeva, Sudhesh Kumar, Charles E. Hutchinson, Thomas M. Barber, 'Identification of brown adipose tissue using MR imaging in a human adult with histological and immunohistochemical confirmation', *Journal of Clinical Endocrinology & Metabolism*, vol. 99, issue 1 (Jan. 2014).

8. Michael E. Symonds, Katrina Henderson, Lindsay Elvidge, Conrad Bosman, Don Sharkey, Alan C. Perkins, Helen Budge, 'Thermal imaging to assess age-related changes of skin temperature within the supraclavicular region co-locating with brown adipose tissue in healthy children', *Journal of Paediatrics*, vol. 161, issue 5 (Nov. 2012).

9. Iain T. H. Au-Yong, Natasha Thorn, Rakesh Ganatra, Alan C. Perkins, Michael E. Symonds, 'Brown adipose tissue and seasonal variations in humans', *Diabetes*, vol. 58, issue 11 (Nov. 2009).

10. Véronique Ouellet, Sébastien M. Labbé, Denis P. Blondin, Serge Phoenix, Brigitte Guérin, François Haman, Eric E. Turcotte, Denis Richard, André C. Carpentier, 'Brown

adipose tissue oxidative metabolism contributes to energy expenditure during acute cold exposure in humans', *Journal of Clinical Investigation*, vol. 122, issue 2 (Feb. 2012).

11. P. Lee, S. Smith, J. Linderman, A. B. Courville, R. J. Brychta, W. Dieckmann, C. D. Werner, K. Y. Chen, F. S. Celi, 'Temperature-acclimated brown adipose tissue modulates insulin sensitivity in humans', *Diabetes* (22 June, 2014) (epub).

12. Pontus Boström, Jun Wu, Mark P. Jedrychowski, Anisha Korde, Li Ye, James C. Lo, Kyle A. Rasbach, Elisabeth Almer Boström, Jang Hyun Choi, Jonathan Z. Long, Shingo Kajimura, Maria Cristina Zingaretti, Birgitte F. Vind, Hua Tu, Saverio Cinti, Kurt Højlund, Steven P. Gygi, Bruce M. Spiegelman, 'A PGC1-α-dependent myokine that drives brown-fat-like development of white fat and thermogenesis', *Nature*, 481 (January 2012).

13. Ippei Shimizu, Tamar Aprahamian, Ryosuke Kikuchi, Ayako Shimizu, Kyriakos N. Papanicolaou, Susan MacLauchlan, Sonomi Maruyama, Kenneth Walsh, 'Vascular rarefaction mediates whitening of brown fat in obesity', *Journal of Clinical Investigation*, vol. 124, issue 5 (May 2014).

14. Megumi Hatori, Christopher Vollmers, Amir Zarrinpar, Luciano DiTacchio, Eric A. Bushong, Shubhroz Gill, Mathias Leblanc, Amandine Chaix, Matthew Joens, James A. J. Fitzpatrick, Mark H. Ellisman, Satchidananda Panda, 'Time-restricted feeding without reducing caloric intake prevents metabolic diseases in mice fed a high-fat diet', *Cell Metabolism*, vol. 15, issue 6 (June 2012).

15. Anne Vrieze, Josefine E. Schopman, Wanda M. Admiraal, Maarten R. Soeters, Max Nieuwdorp, Hein J. Verberne,

Frits Holleman, 'Fasting and postprandial activity of brown adipose tissue in healthy men', *Journal of Nuclear Medicine*, vol. 53, issue 9 (Sept. 2012).

16. S. D. Kunkel, C. J. Elmore, K. S. Bongers, S. M. Ebert, D. K. Fox, Michael C. Dyle, Steven A. Bullard, Christopher M. Adams, 'Ursolic acid increases skeletal muscle and brown fat and decreases diet-induced obesity, glucose intolerance and fatty liver disease', *PLoS One*, vol. 7, issue 6 (June 2012).

17. S. Whiting, E. J. Derbyshire, B. Tiwari, 'Could capsaicinoids help to support weight management? A systematic review and meta-analysis of energy intake data', *Appetite*, 73 (Feb. 2014).

18. Mayumi Yoshioka, Sylvie St-Pierre, Vicky Drapeau, Isabelle Dionne, Eric Doucet, Masashige Suzuki, Angelo Tremblay, 'Effects of red pepper on appetite and energy intake', *British Journal of Nutrition*, vol. 82, issue 2 (Aug. 1999).

19. M. Saito, T. Yoneshiro, 'Capsinoids and related food ingredients activating brown fat thermogenesis and reducing body fat in humans', *Current Opinion in Lipidology*, vol. 24, issue 1 (Feb. 2013).

20. T. Yoneshiro, S. Aita, M. Matsushita, T. Kayahara, T. Kameya, Y. Kawai, T. Iwanaga, M. Saito, 'Recruited brown adipose tissue as an antiobesity agent in humans', *Journal of Clinical Investigation*, vol. 123, issue 8 (August 2013).

21. T. Yoneshiro, S. Aita, Y. Kawai, T. Iwanaga, M. Saito, 'Nonpungent capsaicin analogs (capsinoids) increase energy expenditure through the activation of brown adipose tissue in humans', *American Journal of Clinical Nutrition*, vol. 95, issue 4 (April 2012).

22. Mayumi Yoshioka, Eric Doucet, Vicky Drapeau, Isabelle Dionne, Angelo Tremblay, 'Combined effects of red pepper and caffeine consumption on 24-hour energy balance in subjects given free access to foods', *British Journal of Nutrition*, vol. 85, issue 2 (2001).

23. Michael E. Symonds, Mark Pope, Helen Budge, 'Adipose tissue development during early life: novel insights into energy balance from small and large mammals', *Proceedings of the Nutrition Society*, vol. 71, issue 3 (Aug. 2012).

24. F. Scazzina, D. Del Rio, L. Benini, C. Melegari, N. Pellegrini, E. Marcazzan, F. Brighenti, 'The effects of breakfasts varying in glycaemic index and glycaemic load on dietary induced thermogenesis and respiratory quotient', *Nutrition, Metabolism and Cardiovascular Diseases*, vol. 21, issue 2 (Feb. 2011).

25. K. R. Westerterp, S. A. J. Wilson, V. Rolland, 'Diet Induced Thermogenesis over 24 hr in a respiration chamber: effect of diet composition', *International Journal of Obesity*, vol. 23, issue 3 (March 1999).

26. Thomas F. Hany, Esmaiel Gharehpapagh, Ehab M. Kamel, Alfred Buck, Jean Himms-Hagen, Gustav K. von Schulthess, 'Brown adipose tissue: a factor to consider in symmetrical tracer uptake in the neck and upper chest region', *European Journal of Nuclear Medicine*, vol. 29, issue 10 (Oct. 2002).

27. A. L. Carey, M. F. Formosa, B. Van Every, D. Bertovic, N. Eikelis, G. W. Lambert, V. Kalff, S. J. Duffy, M. H. Cherk, B. A. Kingwell, 'Ephedrine activates brown adipose tissue in lean but not obese humans', *Diabetologia*, vol. 56, issue 1 (Jan. 2013).

28. Aaron M. Cypess, Yih-Chieh Chen, Cathy Sze, Ke Wang, Jeffrey English, Onyee Chan, Ashley R. Holman, Ilan Tal,

Matthew R. Palmer, Gerald M. Kolodny, C. Ronald Kahn, 'Cold but not sympathomimetics activates human brown adipose tissue in vivo', *Proceedings of the National Academy of Sciences of the United States of America*, vol. 109, issue 25 (June 2012).

29. Andrew J. Whittle, Stefania Carobbio, Luís Martins, Marc Slawik, Elayne Hondares, María Jesús Vázquez, Donald Morgan, Robert I. Csikasz, Rosalía Gallego, Sergio Rodriguez-Cuenca, Martin Dale, Samuel Virtue, Francesc Villarroya, Barbara Cannon, Kamal Rahmouni, Miguel López, Antonio Vidal-Puig, 'BMP8B increases brown adipose tissue thermogenesis through both central and peripheral actions', *Cell*, vol. 149, issue 4 (May 2012).

30. Gina Kolata, 'Brown fat, triggered by cold or exercise, may yield a key to weight control', *New York Times*, 24 Jan. 2012.

31. 'Positive effects of brown adipose tissue on femoral bone stucture', *IBMS BoneKEy*, 11, article number 569 (2014).

32. Maria Chondronikola, Elena Volpi, Elisabet Børsheim, Craig Porter, Palam Annamalai, Sven Enerbäck, Martin E. Lidell, Manish K. Saraf, Sebastien M. Labbe, Nicholas M. Hurren, Christina Yfanti, Tony Chao, Clark R. Andersen, Fernardo Cesani, Hal Hawkins, Labros S. Sidossis, 'Brown adipose tissue improves whole body glucose homeostasis and insulin sensitivity in humans', *Diabetes* (23 July 2014) (epub).

33. Patrick Seale, Mitchell A. Lazar, 'Brown fat in humans: Turning up the heat on obesity', *Diabetes*, vol. 58, issue 7 (Jul. 2009).

34. Leontine E. H. Bakker, Mariëtte R. Boon, Rianne A. D. van der Linden, Lenka Pereira Arias-Bouda, Jan B. van Klinken, Frits Smit, Hein J. Verberne, Prof. J. Wouter Jukema, Jouke T.

Tamsma, Prof. Louis M. Havekes, Wouter D. van Marken Lichtenbelt, Ingrid M. Jazet, Prof. Patrick C. N. Rensen, 'Brown adipose tissue volume in healthy lean south Asian adults compared with white Caucasians: a prospective, case-controlled observational study', *The Lancet: Diabetes & Endocrinology*, vol. 2, issue 3 (March 2014).

35. Mei Dong, Xiaoyan Yang, Sharon Lim, Ziquan Cao, Jennifer Honek, Huixia Lu, Cheng Zhang, Takahiro Seki, Kayoko Hosaka, Eric Wahlberg, Jianmin Yang, Lei Zhang, Toste Länne, Baocun Sun, Xuri Li, Yizhi Liu, Yun Zhang, Yihai Cao, 'Cold exposure promotes atherosclerotic plaque growth and instability via UCP1-dependent lipolysis', *Cell Metabolism*, vol. 18, issue 1 (July 2013).

3 The Ice Edge

1. B. C. Weiner, A. C. Weiner, 'The Ice Diet', *Annals of Internal Medicine*, vol. 153, issue 4 (Aug. 2010).

2. M. Boschmann, J. Steiniger, U. Hille, J. Tank, F. Adams, A. M. Sharma, S. Klaus, F. C. Luft, J. Jordan, 'Water-Induced Thermogenesis', *Journal of Clinical Endocrinology and Metabolism*, vol. 88, issue 12 (Dec. 2003).

3. Clive M. Brown, Abdul G. Dulloo, Jean-Pierre Montani, 'Water-induced thermogenesis revisited: The effects of osmolality and water temperature on energy expenditure after drinking', *Journal of Clinical Endocrinology and Metabolism*, vol. 91, issue 9 (Sept. 2006).

4. R. Siegel, J. Maté, M. B. Brearley, G. Watson, K. Nosaka, P. B. Laursen, 'Ice slurry ingestion increases core

temperature capacity and running time in the heat', *Medicine & Science in Sports & Exercise*, vol. 42, issue 4 (April 2010).

5. Jason K. W. Lee, Susan M. Shirreffs, Ronald J. Maughan, 'Cold drink ingestion improves exercise endurance capacity in the heat', *Medicine & Science in Sports & Exercise*, vol. 40, issue 9 (Sept. 2008).

6. Aaron M. Cypess, Yih-Chieh Chen, Cathy Sze, Ke Wang, Jeffrey English, Onyee Chan, Ashley R. Holman, Ilan Tal, Matthew R. Palmer, Gerald M. Kolodny, C. Ronald Kahn, 'Cold but not sympathomimetics activates human brown adipose tissue in vivo', *Proceedings of the National Academy of Sciences of the United States of America*, vol. 109, issue 25 (June 2012).

7. N. J. Crystal, D. H. Townson, S. B. Cook, D. P. LaRoche, 'Effect of cryotherapy on muscle recovery and inflammation following a bout of damaging exercise', *European Journal of Applied Physiology*, vol. 113, issue 10 (Oct. 2013).

8. Chris Bleakley, Suzanne McDonough, Evie Gardner, G. David Baxter, J. T. Hopkins, Gareth W. Davison, 'Cold-water immersion (cryotherapy) for preventing and treating muscle soreness after exercise', *The Cochrane Library* (Feb. 2012) (epub).

4 Users' Manual

1. V. S. Malik, B. M. Popkin, G. A. Bray, J. P. Després, F. B. Hu, 'Sugar-sweetened beverages, obesity, Type 2 diabetes mellitus, and cardiovascular disease risk', *Circulation*, vol. 121, issue 11 (March 2010).

2. Sanjay Basu, Paula Yoffe, Nancy Hills, Robert H. Lustig, 'The relationship of sugar to population-level diabetes prevalence: An econometric analysis of repeated cross-sectional data', *PLoS One*, vol. 8, issue 2 (Feb. 2013).

3. H. J. Leidy, C. L. Armstrong, M. Tang, R. D. Mattes, W. W. Campbell, 'The influence of higher protein intake and greater eating frequency on appetite control in overweight and obese men', *Obesity*, vol. 18, issue 9 (Sep 2010).

4. Hana Kahleova, Lenka Belinova, Hana Malinska, Olena Oliyarnyk, Jaroslava Trnovska, Vojtech Skop, Ludmila Kazdova, Monika Dezortova, Milan Hajek, Andrea Tura, Martin Hill, Terezie Pelikanova, 'Eating two larger meals a day (breakfast and lunch) is more effective than six smaller meals in a reduced-energy regimen for patients with Type 2 diabetes: a randomised crossover study', *Diabetologia*, vol. 57, issue 8 (May 2014).

5. Emily J. Dhurandhar, John Dawson, Amy Alcorn, Lesli H. Larsen, Elizabeth A. Thomas, Michelle Cardel, Ashley C. Bourland, Arne Astrup, Marie-Pierre St-Onge, James O. Hill, Caroline M. Apovian, James M. Shikany, David B. Allison, 'The effectiveness of breakfast recommendations on weight loss: a randomized controlled trial', *American Journal of Clinical Nutrition* (August 2014).

6. James A. Betts, Judith D. Richardson, Enhad A. Chowdhury, Geoffrey D. Holman, Kostas Tsintzas, Dylan Thompson, 'The causal role of breakfast in energy balance and health: a randomized controlled trial in lean adults', *American Journal of Clinical Nutrition* (August 2014).
7. *BBC Good Food Magazine*, September 2014.
8. Marilynn Schnepf, Judy Driskell, 'Sensory attributes and nutrient retention in selected vegetables prepared by conventional and microwave methods', *Journal of Food Quality*, vol. 17, issue 2 (April 1994).

5 Preparing to Acclimatize

1. 'The Big Freeze', National Omnibus Survey conducted by Honeywell Home Heating (Honeywell.com).
2. *The Pop-up Gym*, Jon Denoris, (Bloomsbury, 2014).

6 Getting Ready

1. M. Ashwell, P. Gunn, S. Gibson, 'Waist to height ratio is a better screening tool', *Obesity Reviews*, vol. 13, issue 3 (March 2012).
2. J. G. LaRose, J. Fava, E. Steeves, J. Hecht, R. R. Wing, H. A. Raynor, 'Daily self-weighing within a behavioral weight loss program: Impact on disordered eating symptoms', *Health Psychology*, vol. 33, issue 3 (March 2014).
3. American Council on Exercise.

4. V. Provencher, C. Bégin, A. Tremblay, L. Mongeau, L. Corneau, S. Dodin, S. Boivin, S. Lemieux, 'Health-At-Every-Size and eating behaviours', *Journal of the American Dietetic Association*, vol. 109, issue 11 (Nov. 2009).

7 The 6-Week Ice Diet Plan

Day 5: C. Wagstaff, G. J. J. Clarkson, S. D. Rothwell, A. Page, G. Taylor, M. S. Dixon, 'Characterization of cell death in bagged baby salad leaves', *Postharvest Biology and Technology*, vol. 46, issue 2 (2007).

Day 7: Institute of Food Technologists (IFT), 'The right snack may aid satiety, weight loss', *ScienceDaily* (July 2013).

Day 8: Sharifah S. Syed Alwi, Breeze E. Cavell, Urvi Telang, Marilyn E. Morris, Barbara M. Parry, Graham Packham, 'In vivo modulation of 4E binding protein 1 (4E-BP1) phosphorylation by watercress: a pilot study', *British Journal of Nutrition*, vol. 104, issue 9 (Nov. 2010).

Day 9: V. Er, J. Athene Lane, R. M. Martin, P. Emmett, R. Gilbert, K. N. L. Avery, E. Walsh, J. L. Donovan, D. E. Neal, F. C. Hamdy, M. Jeffreys, 'Adherence to dietary and lifestyle recommendations and prostate cancer risk in the Prostate Testing for Cancer and Treatment (ProtecT) trial', *Cancer Epidemiology Biomarkers & Prevention*, vol. 23, issue 10 (Oct. 2014).

Day 15: H. J. Leidy, L. C. Ortinau, S. M. Douglas, H. A. Hoertel. 'Beneficial effects of a higher-protein breakfast on the appetitive, hormonal, and neural signals controlling energy intake regulation in overweight/obese, "breakfast-skipping" late-adolescent girls', *American Journal of Clinical Nutrition*, vol. 97, issue 4 (April 2013).

Day 16: Gordon J. McDougall, Pat Dobson, Nikki Jordan-Mahy, 'Effect of different cooking regimes on rhubarb polyphenols', *Food Chemistry*, vol. 119, issue 2 (March 2010).

Day 18: Hanna Isaksson, Helena Fredriksson, Roger Andersson, Johan Olsson, Per Åman, 'Effect of rye bread breakfasts on subjective hunger and satiety: a randomized controlled trial', *Nutrition Journal*, vol. 8, issue 39 (Aug. 2009).

Day 20: (1) Katherine E. Lansley, Paul G. Winyard, Stephen J. Bailey, Anni Vanhatalo, Daryl P. Wilkerson, Jamie R. Blackwell, Mark Gilchrist, Nigel Benjamin, Andrew M. Jones, 'Acute dietary nitrate supplementation improves cycling time trial performance', *Medicine & Science in Sports & Exercise*, vol. 43, issue 6 (2011). (2) Tennille D. Presley, Ashley R. Morgan, Erika Bechtold, William Clodfelter, Robin W. Dove, Janine M. Jennings, Robert A. Kraft, S. Bruce King, Paul J. Laurienti, W. Jack Rejeski, 'Acute effect of a high nitrate diet on brain perfusion in older adults', *Nitric Oxide*, vol. 24, issue 1 (Jan. 2011).

Day 23: C. Bosetti, M. Filomeno, P. Riso, J. Polesel, F. Levi, R. Talamini, M. Montella, E. Negri, S. Franceschi, C. La Vecchia, 'Cruciferous vegetables and cancer risk in a network of case-control studies', *Annals of Oncology*, vol. 23, issue 8 (2012).

Day 24: Caroline Montelius, Daniel Erlandsson, Egzona Vitija, Eva-Lena Stenblom, Emil Egecioglu, Charlotte Erlanson-Albertsson, 'Body weight loss, reduced urge for palatable food and increased release of GLP-1 through daily supplementation with green-plant membranes for three months in overweight women', *Appetite*, 81 (Oct. 2014).

Day 25: Anitra C. Carr, Stephanie M. Bozonet, Juliet M. Pullar and Margreet C. M. Vissers, 'Mood improvement in young adult males following supplementation with gold kiwi fruit, a high-vitamin C food', *Journal of Nutritional Science*, vol. 2, e24 (2013).

Day 26: University of Liverpool, 'Eating prunes can help weight loss, study shows', *ScienceDaily* (May 2014).

Day 27: Linda M. Oude Griep, W. M. Monique Verschuren, Daan Kromhout, Marga C. Ocké, Johanna M. Geleijnse, 'Colors of fruit and vegetables and 10-Year Incidence of stroke', *Stroke*, vol. 42 (2011).

Day 29: University of Warwick, 'Boiling broccoli ruins its anti-cancer properties, according to study', *ScienceDaily* (May 2007).

Day 38: Annual Conference of the American Chemical Society 2014, www.acs.org.

9 Ice Exercise

1. Oliver J. Webb and Frank F. Eves, 'Promoting stair climbing: Intervention effects generalize to a subsequent stair ascent', *American Journal of Health Promotion*, vol. 22, issue 2 (Nov./Dec. 2007).

2. Ashley Nereng, John P. Porcari, Clayton Camic, Cordial Gillette, Carl Foster, 'Hot Yoga', ACE *ProSource* (July 2013).

3. Roma Robertson, Ann Robertson, Ruth Jepson, Margaret Maxwell, 'Walking for depression or depressive symptoms:

A systematic review and meta-analysis', *Mental Health and Physical Activity*, vol. 5, issue 1 (June 2012).

4. J. Thomson Koon, K Boddy, K. Stein, R. Whear, J. Barton, M. H. Depledge, 'Does participating in physical activity in outdoor natural environments have a greater effect on physical and mental well-being than physical activity indoors? A systematic review', *Environmental Science and Technology*, vol. 45, issue 5 (March 2011).

5. J. Pretty, J. Peacock, R. Hine, M. Sellens, N. South, M. Griffin, 'Green exercise in the UK countryside: Effects on health and psychological well-being, and implications for policy and planning', *Journal of Environmental Planning and Management*, vol. 50, issue 2 (March 2007).

6. P. G. Weyand, B. R. Smith, M. R. Puyau, N. F. Butte, 'The mass-specific energy cost of human walking is set by stature', *Journal of Experimental Biology*, vol. 213, pt. 23 (Dec. 2010).

7. Rebecca Scalzo, Garrett Peltonen, Gregory Giordano, Scott Binns, Anna Klochak, Hunter Paris, Melani Schweder, Steve Szallar, Lacey Wood, Dennis Larson, Gary Luckasen, Matthew Hickey, Christopher Bell, 'Regulators of human white adipose browning: evidence for control and sexual dimorphic response to sprint interval training', *PLoS One*, vol. 9, issue 3 (March 2014).

8. Dr Michael Mosley and Peta Bee, *Fast Exercise* (Short Books, 2013).

9. K. A. Burgomaster, K. R. Howarth, S. M. Phillips, M. Rakobowchuk, M. J. Macdonald, S. L. McGee, M. J. Gibala, 'Similar metabolic adaptations during exercise after low volume sprint interval training and traditional endurance

training in humans', *Journal of Physiology*, vol. 586, issue 1 (Jan. 2008).

10. J. Jakeman, S. Adamson, J. Babraj, 'Extremely short duration high-intensity training substantially improves endurance performance in triathletes', *Applied Physiology, Nutrition, and Metabolism*, vol. 37, issue 5 (Oct. 2012).

11. Brett Klika, Chris Jordan, 'High intensity circuit training using body weight: maximum results with minimum effort', *ACSM's Health and Fitness Journal*, vol. 17, issue 13 (May/ June 2013).

12. Arnt Erik Tjønna, Ingeborg Megaard Leinan, Anette Thoresen Bartnes, Bjørn M. Jenssen, Martin J. Gibala, Richard A. Winett, Ulrik Wisløff, 'Low and high volume of intensive endurance training significantly improves maximal oxygen uptake after 10 weeks of training in healthy men', *PLoS One*, vol. 8, issue 5 (May 2013).

13. V. Mougios, A. Deligiannis, 'Effect of water temperature on performance, lactate production and heart rate at swimming of maximal and submaximal intensity', *Journal of Sports Medicine and Physical Fitness*, vol. 33, issue 1 (March 1993).

14. Swimming Pool Temperatures, www.britishswimming.org.

Acknowledgements

This book would not have been possible without the many scientists and researchers who were willing to spend much of their valuable time talking and corresponding with me about their work. In particular I'd like to thank:

Michael Symonds, Professor of Developmental Physiology, Faculty of Medicine & Health Sciences, University of Nottingham, for introducing me to the concept of 'good' fat and allowing me access to trials in his labs.

Ray Cronise of Thermogenex and hypothermics.com, who is a true scientific trailblazer and whose expertise in the area of 'cooling' and its effects on the human body is second to none.

Jamie Timmons, Professor of Systems Biology at Kings College, University of London, who has helped me to unravel some of the complex science relating to exercise and the activation (or not) of brown fat as well as the importance of HIIT.

Dr Brian Weiner, Marlboro Gastro, New Jersey, for discussing his innovative 'ical' theories.

Professor Mike Cawthorne, Director of Metabolic Research, Head of the School of Medicine, University of Buckingham, for his expert opinions on heating in homes.

ACKNOWLEDGEMENTS

Paul Strzelecki, Honorary Visiting Professor at the University of Manchester, for his assistance with sourcing some of the latest 'ice' technologies.

John Brewer, Professor of Applied Sport Science at St Mary's University, Twickenham, for his help with all things exercise-related.

He just wanted a decent book to read ...

Not too much to ask, is it? It was in 1935 when Allen Lane, Managing Director of Bodley Head Publishers, stood on a platform at Exeter railway station looking for something good to read on his journey back to London. His choice was limited to popular magazines and poor-quality paperbacks – the same choice faced every day by the vast majority of readers, few of whom could afford hardbacks. Lane's disappointment and subsequent anger at the range of books generally available led him to found a company – and change the world.

'We believed in the existence in this country of a vast reading public for intelligent books at a low price, and staked everything on it'
Sir Allen Lane, 1902–1970, founder of Penguin Books

The quality paperback had arrived – and not just in bookshops. Lane was adamant that his Penguins should appear in chain stores and tobacconists, and should cost no more than a packet of cigarettes.

Reading habits (and cigarette prices) have changed since 1935, but Penguin still believes in publishing the best books for everybody to enjoy. We still believe that good design costs no more than bad design, and we still believe that quality books published passionately and responsibly make the world a better place.

So wherever you see the little bird – whether it's on a piece of prize-winning literary fiction or a celebrity autobiography, political tour de force or historical masterpiece, a serial-killer thriller, reference book, world classic or a piece of pure escapism – you can bet that it represents the very best that the genre has to offer.

Whatever you like to read – trust Penguin.